True to Form

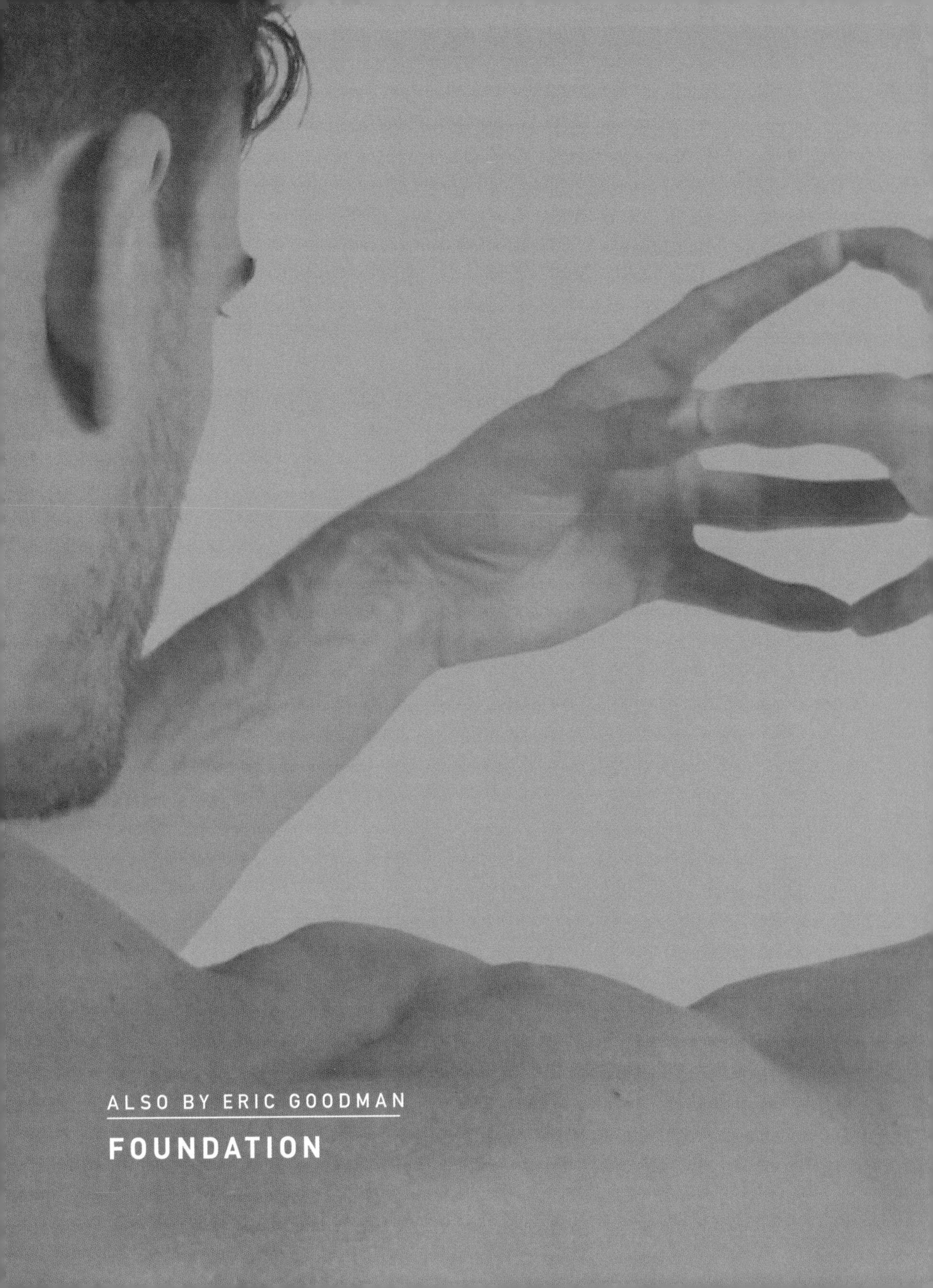

ALSO BY ERIC GOODMAN

FOUNDATION

True to Form

How to Use Foundation Training
for Sustained Pain Relief
and Everyday Fitness

Dr. Eric Goodman

HARPER WAVE

An Imprint of HarperCollinsPublishers

HarperCollins books may be purchased for educational, business, or sales promotional use. For information, please e-mail the Special Markets Department at SPsales@harpercollins.com.

FIRST EDITION

Designed by William Ruoto

Photographs by David Nehmer and the team at Noble

Illustrations by Justin Kleiner and Dr. Dustin DeRyke

Library of Congress Cataloging-in-Publication Data has been applied for.

ISBN: 978-0-06-231531-1

16 17 18 19 20   OV/RRD   10 9 8 7 6 5 4 3 2 1

TO GOODMANS, FORRESTS, BLUMS,
AND BLOOMS.

ALSO TO FOUNDATION TRAINING INSTRUCTORS
AROUND THE WORLD.

AND SPECIFICALLY TO KAREN RINALDI,
WITH A LOT OF APPRECIATION.

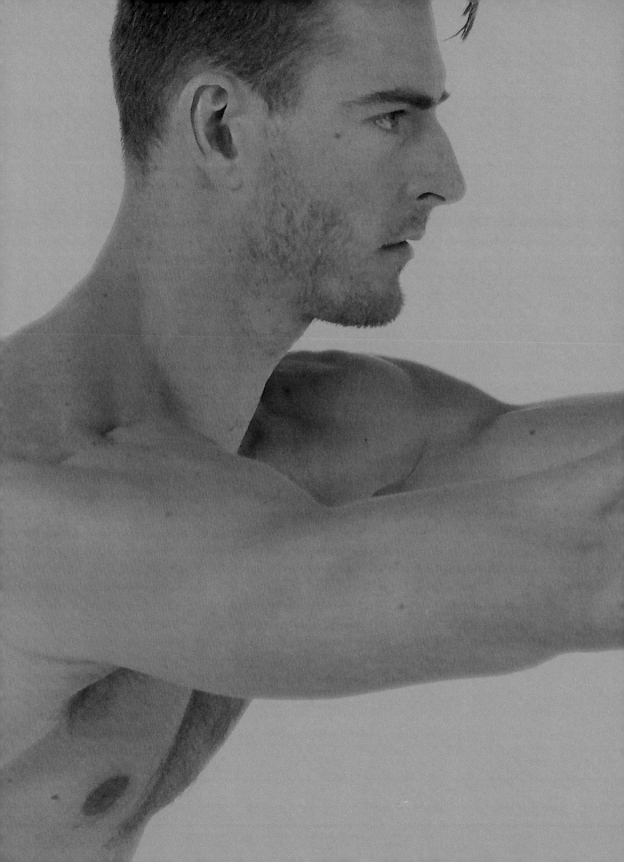

EVERYONE IS BORN A GENIUS,

BUT THE PROCESS OF LIVING

DE-GENIUSES THEM.

—R. BUCKMINSTER FULLER

CONTENTS

Part III: Sustained Pain Relief and Everyday Fitness

FOREWORD

Until I started doing Foundation Training, I couldn't lift Thor's hammer—at least, not without help from Hollywood magic. The problem was that I had injured my back while shooting a movie a few years ago, and it had gotten progressively worse. I tried all sorts of rehab and strengthening programs, stretching, isolated muscle-building, and more, but nothing ever gave me a long-term benefit. I was alternating between limiting my exercises in order to heal the injury and doing more exercises in order to strengthen my back where it felt vulnerable.

Then a stuntman on a film I was working on told me about Foundation Training. He had seriously injured his back, and it was FT that had paved the way to his recovery. I decided to try it. What did I have to lose? I'd tried just about everything else.

I began with some of the workout videos available online. The benefits were immediately noticeable. Over the coming months, as I began working one-on-one with Eric, my back grew stronger than ever. For the first time in years, I felt combined flexibility and strength in places that had previously been incredibly vulnerable.

Today I do a Foundation Training sequence four or five times a week for maintenance—and whenever my back feels overworked, tight, or painful. I'm now able to do all the activities I did in the past with confidence; I don't have to baby myself through any particular movements. I've also learned, under Eric's guidance, how to restructure my movement patterns and do away with bad habits that could lead to further trouble—worse trouble.

Like that stuntman, like so many people who have found relief from pain with Foundation Training, I am grateful for the healing. I am even more grateful for having learned how to fully engage my true core muscles so as to keep my body at peak strength and flexibility. That is the true gift of Foundation Training, and it is the message at the heart of this book.

—CHRIS HEMSWORTH

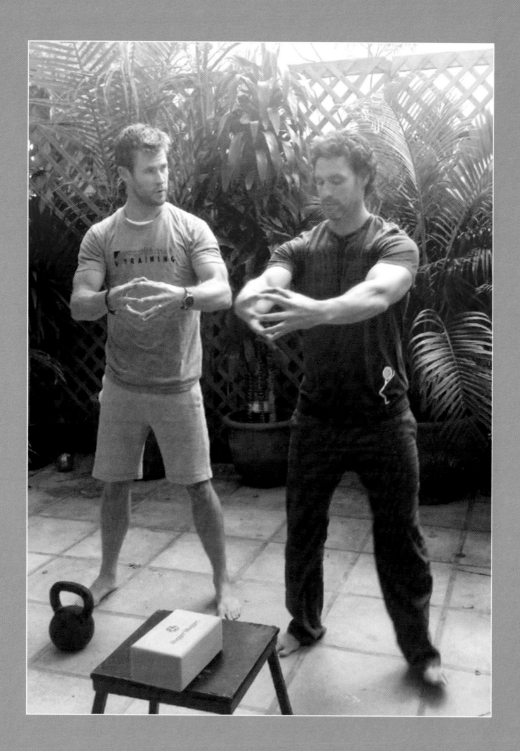

INTRODUCTION

FROM PAIN TO
PERFORMANCE

When I was fifteen years old, I had surgery to repair my right shoulder joint. The procedure was over in a couple of hours, but the recovery took forever. For the next six weeks—an eternity at that age—I had to wear a gigantic white brace that lashed my right arm tight to my body with Velcro. I wore the brace in school and after school, day and night, and when it finally came off, my arm was a noodle. It took another six months before I was able to play the sports I loved at all, and it took much longer to feel comfortable playing.

It was an awful experience, although I think it was one of the reasons that I decided to make chiropractic medicine my profession, and shortly after college, I enrolled in a graduate program and began my training.

Three years into it—in fact, not too long before I was to graduate and launch my career—doctors were recommending I go under the knife again—this time for chronic back pain that had very nearly immobilized me. Those of you who know the reality of chronic back pain and are familiar with the lingo will understand when I say that my MRI showed substantial degeneration of the fourth and fifth lumbar vertebrae and of the sacrum at the base of the spine. My bottom two vertebrae, the L5 and S1, were actually sitting one on top of the other, which pretty much explained why I could barely move so much of the time. For years I had been treating the symptoms—the pain—with increasingly potent and varied painkillers, along with physical therapy, chiropractic adjustments, and the typical forms of rehab that were available at that time. But there was no progress; nothing was fixed. Worse, my pain was no longer responding to the drugs, and the potential side effects and interactions were becoming their own health issue. The only recourse now, recommended by a team of highly trained specialists, was fusion surgery, a major procedure in which bone would be grafted onto my spine to fuse the two problem vertebrae, stop the motion between the two, and, if it all worked, alleviate the pain.

I was twenty-six. Eleven years after the shoulder operation had incapacitated me for half a year, "major surgery" was about the last thing I wanted to hear.

I was also aware of the irony of the situation, which was painful in a different way. I was about to enter a profession aimed precisely at helping patients find healing outside of surgery, yet I was unable to find such healing for myself. "Up-and-Coming Young Chiropractor Undergoes Back Surgery" is not a good headline for someone starting a career dedicated to preventing others from having to go under the knife for their back pain.

Mostly, I could not fathom how I had gotten here. I was young, strong, athletic. Why was my body being shut down by physical pain? What was the reason my twenty-six-year-old discs were as worn and torn as ninety-six-year-old ones—maybe more so?

Moreover, I wasn't just a random guy who played sports and worked out in a gym; I was someone who studied how the body worked, a student of the musculoskeletal system and its interactions with the other systems of human physiology. What had I missed? Why had I failed to apprehend what was happening to me while it was happening so that I could catch it, stop it, and turn it back around?

I decided I needed to understand all this far more than I needed surgery. It took some time and much trial and error, but in the process I recognized something so fundamental, so essentially obvious that it has taken me a decade of practice and study to sort it out.

We move wrong.

More specifically, we move in ways contrary to how our bodies are naturally constructed and equipped for us to move. Many of us endure chronic pain precisely because we do not understand how to live correctly inside the efficiently designed bodies we are born into. We weren't given an operating manual and for some reason, our instincts have failed us.

This book sets out to change all that.

It all starts with the bodies we have and what we're doing to them.

PART ONE

Off Your Form and Under Pressure

ONE

A DAY IN THE LIFE OF A TWENTY-FIRST-CENTURY BODY

Meet Hallie.

She works for a large company in a large office—work she loves—and like so many of us, she is consigned to a desk for the greater part of every workday. Atop her desk is a bank of computer monitors on which Hallie tracks and manages a range of projects, procedures, and operational activities. She does it all sitting down, although often on the very edge of her high-tech, lumbar-supported, mesh-backed, spongy-seat office chair, as she peers with acute concentration at first one screen, then another. Hallie typically rests her elbows or forearms on the desk or her lap, and her hands and wrists on her computer keyboard. Her body's spine is curved toward her work,

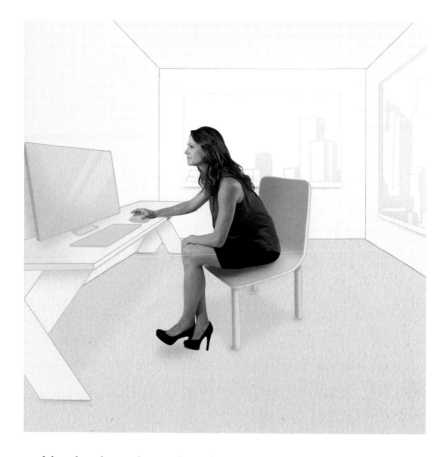

and her head juts forward as if it wanted to be ready to meet the next piece of vital information head-on.

It's a common posture for people who work in offices, and here's what it does to Hallie—and to you, if you're in a similar situation.

Since her legs don't have to hold her up, Hallie's lower back does the job instead, becoming the weight-bearing center of her body, which is not what the lower back was designed to be. She feels the consequences of that discrepancy in a recurring back pain, which is getting worse. She also feels tension in her neck, no doubt because

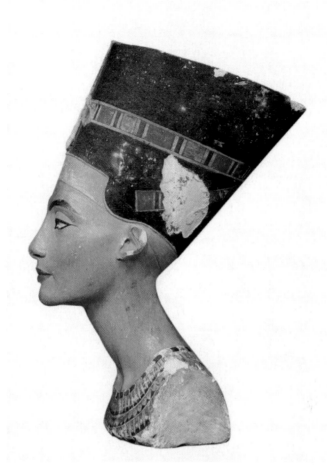

her normal workday posture thrusts her head so far forward that she overextends and stresses her neck muscles.

It's called anterior head carriage (sometimes also known as lollipop head), and while it may have looked good on Queen Nefertiti in the famous bust in the Neues Museum in Berlin—of course, Nefertiti's head had to hold up the enormous, elongated crown of Egypt—it's really a shortening of the muscles at the back of the skull, the occiput, in a misalignment that strains the neck. No wonder Hallie longs for a masseur to knead the back of her neck at the end of every workday. She suffers from headaches too, and she routinely takes aspirin or ibuprofen to alleviate them.

But these standard, garden-variety aches and pains—after all, 80 percent of American adults complain of back pain—are just the beginning of what's happening to Hallie, the tip of an iceberg of disasters that derive from the simple fact that in the life she lives, resisting gravity is something she does rarely and in minor ways, even though her body is built to resist gravity repeatedly and in myriad ways.

Because Hallie does not resist gravity sufficiently, gravity compresses her. The muscles constructed to keep her upright against gravity have weakened from lack of use; the joints taking the pressure the muscles *should* absorb have grown rigid. That's backward from the way things should work, leaving Hallie with weak muscles and stiff joints—the exact opposite of what they should be.

As a result, Hallie's chest droops downward under the force of gravity, taking her ribcage with it and pressing the ribcage into her pelvis, thereby shortening her torso and further bending the muscles of her lower back out of shape. Inside this drooping structure, everything gets squashed, flattened, jammed together in a body that is pressed forward, collapsed inward, squeezed down, out of alignment, and off-balance. That's what compression by gravity does, and it is the daily condition of Hallie's life.

The consequences of this compression—apart from the aches and pains in Hallie's back, neck, and head? They influence every system, process, and function of her physiology.

Start with her breathing. Hallie's lungs—everybody's lungs—are protected by the ribcage, which, powered by the muscles around it, expands and contracts to make breathing happen. Compress the ribcage and the muscles around it cannot expand and contract to the full—and neither can the lungs. Hallie's breathing is diminished: less oxygen in, less carbon dioxide out, and too much residual stuff left over in the lower lobes of the lungs.

Impeded breathing, of course, shortchanges everything else. It can disrupt or obstruct any or all of the functions and activities Hallie's organs are there to carry out; such disruptions are at the heart of most of the chronic illnesses that plague us today. It can slow Hallie's metabolism. It can create a self-perpetuating pattern of pain. Moreover, respiration is at the root of immunity; cheat your breathing and you cheat your body's ability to protect itself from toxic influences. Hallie gets a lot of colds.

Compression that squashes Hallie's torso affects her digestion too. For one thing, it reduces the space available for the digestive process and therefore for the body's ability to obtain nourishment from what she eats. It also affects the enteric nervous system, the body's so-called second brain, or brain in the gut, that part of the central nervous system that resides in and controls the gastrointestinal system and, with its network of neurotransmitters, sends and receives messages to and from all parts of the body. This second brain also serves a major role in Hallie's sense of well-being, and it is not uncommon for Hallie to feel out of sorts in general and to attribute it to what she refers to as "a nervous stomach."

Compression affects her posterior chain of muscles—consisting of her aching lower back muscles, the gluteal muscles of the butt she tries to keep taut through marathon Spinning bike sessions, and the hamstrings and calves that routinely dangle beneath her fashionable desk chair. Compression of this posterior chain causes a breakdown of movement that snowballs across Hallie's body, for these are the muscles that transfer force so you can move your body forward and, by the same token, keep it upright and stable. Precisely because she sits all day and therefore is not activating the posterior chain to do what it was built to do, Hallie is at a mechanical disadvantage when she needs the muscles for forward movement, or for stability, or for being upright. That mechanical disadvantage has made it almost impossible for Hallie to lift her young son anymore; the muscles for that are effectively out of action through lack of use. Instead, her joints and spine have taken the pressure and stiffened up in response, and Hallie swears she can feel the creaking whenever she bends down to reach for her boy or turns her head when he calls.

Even her central nervous system—fundamental control center of the body's functions—is affected by the compression inflicted on Hallie by the way she lives. The system consists of the brain and the spinal cord, which is located inside the spinal column and serves as a transport canal or highway. It is in fact the main highway between the brain, which controls everything in the body, and the periphery of the body—arms, legs, and skin. Dense electric fibers travel up and down the spinal-cord highway to and from the brain. The fibers carry messages of sensory stimuli and motor response, both voluntary and involuntary, back and forth through all the pathways of the body, branching and weaving as needed to get the right response to the right part of the body, then to carry the follow-up message back to the brain, constantly.

When the spine is compressed—especially when the pressure falls on the thickest part of the nerves closer to the spinal cord—the output for motor response becomes less efficient. When the motor output is less efficient, the follow-up sensory input is likewise less efficient. When both the sensory and the motor pathways are less efficient, the entire system becomes less efficient, and that in turn can cause an imbalance in whatever vital process the system handles—digestion and elimination, respiration, immunity, energy, etc. To top it off, most such imbalances occur right at the intersecting points of the weblike, branching formations of neural pathways known as nerve plexuses, bundles of intertwined nerves that branch off the spine and control a substantial portion of the body's functions. The result is a less-than-optimal working order for Hallie's entire body, as all interconnected communication systems get thrown off message and further exacerbate the imbalances affecting the organs and the physiological processes that should keep her body in working order. It's something Hallie can't see or quite define, but it's there nevertheless.

Her Nefertiti neck makes the situation even worse.

It's all about the vagus nerve, the longest of the twelve cranial nerves, and one of the longest nerve systems in the body—the name means "wandering." Among other things, the vagus nerve commands such involuntary body processes as heart rate and the movement of

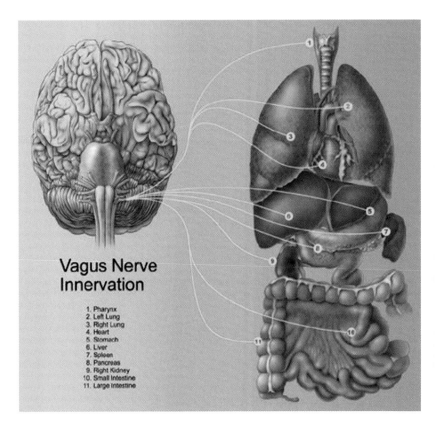

The vagus nerve needs space to communicate the data messages traveling from the organs to the brain.

the muscles that keep us breathing as well as regulation of the chemical levels in the digestive system. You don't want your vagus nerve to get squeezed and affect those functions adversely, but that's what can happen when the head is thrust forward and the neck muscles are shortened—the anterior head carriage position that virtually defines Hallie's profile when she is hard at work.

As to those ills she *can* define—especially her weakening back and all that tenseness in the neck—Hallie tends to fight them by heading for the gym and putting her body through a fairly demanding fitness workout including Spin cycling, strength training, and weight lifting. She is a passionate performer of crunches—her way of strengthening the bad back—and she is sure the weight lifting keeps her body lean. Maybe. But any engineer will tell you that adding a load onto a structure that is already out of balance is a surefire way to weaken the structure further till it eventually breaks down, and the same is true of the human body. And since Hallie's posterior chain muscles are already weak through lack of use, strengthening her *anterior* muscles through crunches just exacerbates that weakness. Hallie keeps making her workout tougher so she can get fitter, and her washboard abs are impressive, but she's further diminishing her body's ability to hold a strong posture to push back against gravity. Her intensity aggravates her aching back and neck, and the vague discomfort in many of her joints and limbs. Her workout helps her mind, but it harms her body. This does not have to be.

WE ARE ALL HALLIE

The problem is that in the advanced industrial societies of the twenty-first century, just about all of us are Hallie.

We spend most of our time seated behind the wheel of a car, or in front of a computer screen at work, or poised over our smartphones or tablets as we text and email, or chilling out in front of the television in the evening, or all of the above. This is our norm, the bonus we have gained because we live in societies that spare us the need to do backbreaking physical labor day after day in order to earn our daily bread or put a roof over our heads or gain security for our families.

The upshot is that we have relegated muscles designed to push back against gravity and support our frames to minor roles that ask little of them. Unengaged, those muscles end up collapsing inward onto our joints as compression squashes our bodies, leaving it to the joints to hold us up. That's a job the joints don't do very well because they were built for an entirely different purpose—namely, to be the flexible, hinging intersections between bones. What it comes down to is that we're out of sync with our own bodies, or rather, our bodies are out of sync with what they were designed to do. We are living in a way that is at odds with how our bodies were engineered.

Worse, our bodies have adapted to this discordance—I call it "complacent adaptation"—which modifies into compression. The modifications manifest themselves as chronic lifestyle complaints, persistent weakness, limitations on our activities, and recurring and ever-worsening illnesses—all of which we alleviate, but do not fundamentally fix. Moving wrong—and suffering for it—is the state of our lives and the state of our bodies in the twenty-first century.

COMPRESSION, CHRONIC ILLNESS, AND THE MEDICAL RESPONSE

And how does our health-care system respond to this dire situation? Typically, it does so by suggesting we take a pill, or get a shot, or have invasive surgery. Brilliant when it comes to critical care, medical practice today seems confused in dealing with the debilitating chronic ailments—body aches and pains but also disorders of respiration, digestion, brain function, locomotion, even mood—that now dominate the health landscape.

There's a reason this is the case. In its genius for specialization, our health-care system has encouraged researchers and practitioners alike to perfect their expertise in separate and distinct areas of concentration. Yes, "miracle" cures have been one result of this, but at the cost of a whole-body systems approach to health care. Chronic illnesses, however, by nature produce symptoms each of which is but a fragmentary message; putting together the fragments to see the whole picture of causation requires just such a whole-body systems approach. And while practitioners today are increasingly—and encouragingly— paying more attention to such an approach, for the most part symptoms are still what gets treated.

Patients and doctors alike tend to look upon every ache as a fresh problem from a cause we haven't experienced before. Neck pain is seen as both distinct and distant from, say, a digestive order. After all, how could there possibly be a connection? It is quicker and may even appear more compassionate to alleviate a patient's suffering with one or some of the many treatments available: pills for the headaches and tension in the neck, injections for the backaches and knee pain, and surgery when the bad back becomes so painful and debilitating it limits your life.

The problem is that the relief, if any, is temporary at best, for the pill and the shot and the operation have targeted only a single effect of what is actually a multifaceted cause encompassing numerous connected parts. Even worse, as our bodies adapt to the relief—bodies are almost infinitely adaptable—we need another but stronger pill, another but higher-dose injection, maybe even another surgical procedure. With each iteration of response to the symptom, our bodies are dragged even further away from addressing the original cause; they adjust to the "cure" without our ever confronting the "disease."

But confronting it means only returning our bodies to their natural postures—something we can do on our own, a fundamental form of self-care. It means relearning how to hold ourselves structurally and how to move muscularly in the way the body was built to be held and to move.

The fact is that our physiology, whether sitting, standing, or on the move, is ideally suited to push back against gravity—and in so doing, to decompress, unfurl, and elongate jammed bodies and experience all the vital power and flexibility of which those bodies are inherently capable. The solution for this modern plague of compression goes right back to the basics of how our bodies work, which is why I call it Foundation Training.

TWO

DESIGNED FOR EFFICIENT

MOVEMENT

What are the basics of that physiology so well suited to resisting gravity? What is the foundational structural design that contemporary lifestyles have weakened—simply because the lifestyles discourage or in some cases prevent us from engaging the design in all its potential? To answer those questions, we need to look back to the late Pleistocene era, which began some 250,000 years ago and ended about 12,000 years ago—for that is when the bodies bequeathed to you and me and Hallie were evolutionarily perfected.

The physiology achieved by Pleistocene humans was perfectly suited to their nomadic, foraging lives, which consisted of nearly constant movement in order to find, obtain, and prepare food. Paleontologists surmise that Pleistocene men and women were upright and on the move for most daylight hours, walking and/or running from five to ten miles per day.

Their posture—that is, the way they held themselves structurally and the way they moved muscularly—fitted that need: Movement was initiated at the hip joint, the body's natural pivot point and therefore the most efficient and effective way to launch oneself into action; torsos were extended and sternums high to accommodate the breathing that filled the lungs sufficiently to power the needed movement; and the body was elongated so these hunter-gatherers could see as far as possible from atop long, straight necks while being supported from the arches of their feet upward. Possessing a structural integrity that could deliver stability and flexibility in equal measure, the body could be held in balance and moved for maximum results for a relatively minimal expenditure of energy. These structural attributes produced a survival differential significant enough to win the reproduction lottery down through the generations. Codified in our DNA, the structure has been the foundation of human physiology ever since.

In the twenty-first century, to be sure, except for a dwindling handful of people, we do not live as hunter-gatherers. We are not on the move all day; in fact, the contrary is the more likely scenario—witness Hallie. But we still inhabit the body structure perfected long ago, designed for balance and efficiency, stability and flexibility.

THE BODY'S STRUCTURAL INTEGRITY

The design begins in the bony framework of the structure, the skeleton, and in the muscles that pull the bones and make the structure move. It isn't easy to push aside the mental picture, beloved of cartoonists, of the wired skeleton found in the traditional anatomy classroom, or to strip our imaginations of the notion that muscles somehow hang off the skeleton and draw bones together as they contract. In reality, of course, there are no metal wires inside us, and muscles don't hang. Rather, the body is one living, interconnected network: a frame of bones connected in ways that enable movement, muscles that carry energy and convert it into power to both move the frame and hold it still, connective tissue, and an enveloping biological fabric, the fascia—within which numerous related organic systems execute the essential processes of life.

The bony skeleton actually consists of two parts: the axial skeleton and the appendicular skeleton. The axial skeleton runs from the head to the sacrum—minus the shoulders—and includes the skull, spine, ribcage, and the sacrum itself, lodged at the midpoint of the pelvis between the hip bones. The appendicular skeleton consists of the shoulders, arms and legs, feet, and pelvis, including the hips.

Axial and appendicular are not opposed to one another; rather, they are and should always be in a state of what we might call competitive tension. That tension is essential to the structural integrity of the body and exemplifies a core paradigm of the body's structural design—namely, the push-pull built into the biomechanics of the

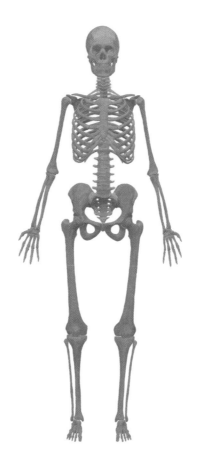

The Axial Skeleton (blue) is made up of the entire vertebral column, sacrum, coccyx, skull, and ribcage. **The Appendicular Skeleton** (gray) is made up of the limbs, scapula, and pelvis. Remember that that pelvis is part of the appendicular skeleton.

body's structure. The most basic push-pull of the design begins at birth and never stops: It is the natural pushback of our body's structure against the downward pull of gravity that would otherwise press us quite literally toward the center of the earth. But for the push-pull between the axial skeleton and the appendicular skeleton, the metaphor I like to use is hot-air ballooning, with the balloon (and basket) in the role of the axial skeleton and the tether attached to the ground serving as the appendicular skeleton.

For the balloon to rise, which is its purpose, it must constantly expand upward and outward. It needs "lift" to get and stay aloft. Similarly, the axial skeleton, and in particular the bones of the ribcage, need expansion for their purpose—which is to house and protect the lungs—and they get it through muscular contraction. Expansion through contraction sounds like a contradiction, but the way it works is that muscles pull, contracting from long to short, and that contracting action expands the bones of the ribcage the muscles support, enabling the ribcage to fill out and lift to serve its protective purpose.

Central to this process is that as the sternum lifts and expands outwardly, the action expands the shoulders as well, an expansion that consists in the shoulders rotating externally in the shoulder joints—the left and right glenohumeral joints. It's a subtle, gentle rotation; in a sense, the front of the shoulder moves expansively while the back of the shoulder contracts. But subtle and gentle as it is, because the upper arm that the joint controls is its own weight, this external rotation represents the shoulder's sustained resistance to gravity. The sum total of axial expansion, therefore, is that the skeleton extends outward and upward, the sternum lifts, and the upper extremities rotate externally—giving the lungs room to breathe and supporting the head and neck against the force of gravity. (As Hallie showed us, if the rotation goes in the other direction—inward—the shoulders droop, the

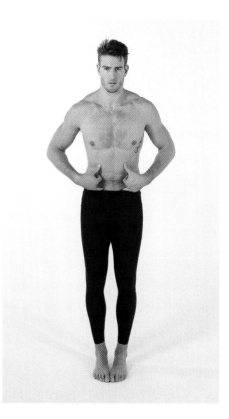

The body can become a burdensome load to carry. Subtle, compressed postures alter the way the body supports itself.

sternum can't expand fully, and the head and neck flop, with numerous adverse impacts on health and well-being.)

Axial expansion rules; it is protective of the brain and breathing and is therefore absolutely vital for a healthy life. The appendicular skeleton, the rope that keeps the balloon from flying away, is essential for support of axial expansion. It does the job through counter-rotation

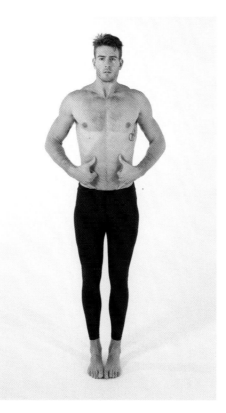

A decompressed torso, versus the compressed torso in the picture opposite, significantly changes the carriage of the shoulders, chest, abdomen, and neck. These changes can be felt throughout the whole body.

that resists the lift of the axial skeleton. Internal rotation at the pelvis, assisted by collaborative pulls from muscles on the inside of the pelvic wings and along the inside of the thighs—respectively, iliacus and adductors—holds in place the gluteal muscles of the backside and the posterior chain of muscles supporting the spine. From the arches of the feet to the pubic symphysis, the muscles supporting the appendic-

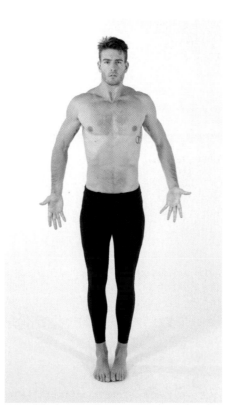

Train the muscles on the back of the torso with isometric poses like those found in Foundation Training to build the endurance to maintain an expansive torso.

ular skeleton—along the legs and in the shoulders—pull upward and inward. In holding the lifting balloon to its position, they support and enable its purpose.

The two parts of the body's skeletal framework need one another: To provide tethering support successfully, the appendicular skeleton needs an expansive axial skeleton; to expand sternum and shoulders, the axial skeleton requires a strongly anchored appendicular skeleton.

Lift and resistance, expansion and contraction, inward against outward rotation: The push-pull tension between the two parts of the framework keeps all of the moving parts of the body in the right place, keeps us upright, keeps us stable enough not to fall over in a slight breeze and flexible enough to bend when the slight breeze turns into a stiff wind.

WHERE MOVEMENT BEGINS

Significantly, the anchoring core of the skeletal structure is precisely at the point where the axial skeleton and the appendicular skeleton meet, just where the hip bones join together at the bottom of the sacrum, directly above the coccyx or tailbone. This is the pubic symphysis and it is the body's center of gravity. You can locate it on your body approximately five inches below the navel, which people used to think of as the center of the body, or three fingers below the navel if you use the measurement of Japanese martial arts practitioners. They refer to the spot as the *hara*, the vital center of the self.

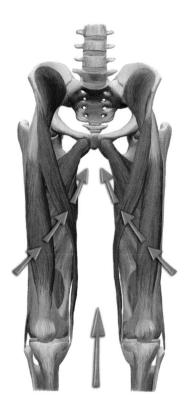

Anchoring musculature pulls upward toward the pubic symphysis (the point which securely fastens the two halves of the pelvis) from various angles. Their collaborative effort yields a strong and stable center of gravity.

The pubic symphysis is also the pivot point from which movement is optimally initiated, optimally both for the movement being executed—standing, walking, bending, reaching, squatting, lifting, anything other than sitting—and for the overall stability, flexibility, and indeed health of the whole body. The most efficient and effective movement the body can execute happens here, in the pelvis, from the muscles supporting the hip joint. When it's time to apply force against gravity—to shift position, to turn, or to hinge—this is the place to start.

SPACE TO COMMUNICATE, ROOM TO SPARE

Controlling every single one of these actions is the brain, the organ that constantly receives sensory input signals from around the entire ecosystem of the body, then transmits responses—in the form of chemical reactions, instructions for cell repair or growth, needed nutrients—to its farthest and deepest regions across a highly complex network. As engineered back in the Pleistocene era, that network begins with a spacious spinal cord providing a wide corridor for transmissions to and from the brain—sensory input in, motor output out. The corridor then expands into almost endlessly branching and weaving pathways along which energy transfer junctions redirect the traffic of neural transmitters so each is dispatched to the right location. Essential to the smooth working of the network is space—room to spare for the traffic of transmissions, and space around the neurological input and output points so that the dispatching, the branching, and the weaving can proceed smoothly, in unimpeded fashion.

The more room there is, the smoother the flow. The smoother the flow, the more efficient and effective the communications. The more efficient the communications, the more capable the body is to turn on a dime in responding to shifting environmental conditions or opportunities—the need to convert fuel to energy, to feel fear or pain, to run or reach.

How does the body maintain the space within for all the transmitters of messages and transporters of nutrients? By holding itself structurally as long and wide as possible. Fossil evidence shows that although our Pleistocene ancestors were considerably shorter in stature than modern humans, they maintained long bodies. Their torsos were elongated the whole length of the spine from top to bottom, from skull to pubic symphysis. This not only makes room to spare in the space within the body; it also stabilizes the spine and the posterior chain of muscles supporting it so that the hips can move easily. Pleistocene man and woman also breathed big—they needed lots of breath to fuel all that walking and running—by lifting and expanding their ribcage front and back, while the muscles supporting their appendicular skeleton stayed long through pulling the skeleton upward. The result was that the individual's natural posture, his or her at-rest position, was a bodily structure designed for efficient movement and at all times ready and equipped to respond to the slightest asymmetry in the environment.

BACK TO THE FUTURE—OR AHEAD TO THE PAST?

That was all a long while ago. The times and circumstances changed. So did patterns of movement—from the agricultural revolution, which meant that our more recent ancestors no longer had to be on the move all day to find food, through the industrial revolution, which sat people down in factories to execute repetitive movements all day long, to today's high-tech era and the lifestyle, exemplified by Hallie.

What has not fundamentally changed is the physiology of the human body. It took hundreds of thousands of years to fine-tune that physiology, so it is unlikely to change substantively in a mere fourteen thousand or so. That means we still possess the physical capabilities for efficient and effective movement for which our contemporary way of life seems to have little need. We've allowed those capabilities to wither through neglect, and the consequences have been both painful and deleterious to our health.

It stands to reason that if we can return our bodies to the physiological foundation we all started out with, we can recover the capabilities the foundation promised and perhaps reverse the adverse effects of the neglect. That is the aim of Foundation Training, and it works in two ways: one, through decompression movements that unwind and elongate the body to release the pent-up pressures of a body that has insufficiently resisted gravity; and two, through anchoring movements that strengthen the body's ability to hold itself upright and propel itself with stability and flexibility through various planes and axes of movement.

PART TWO

Return
to
Form

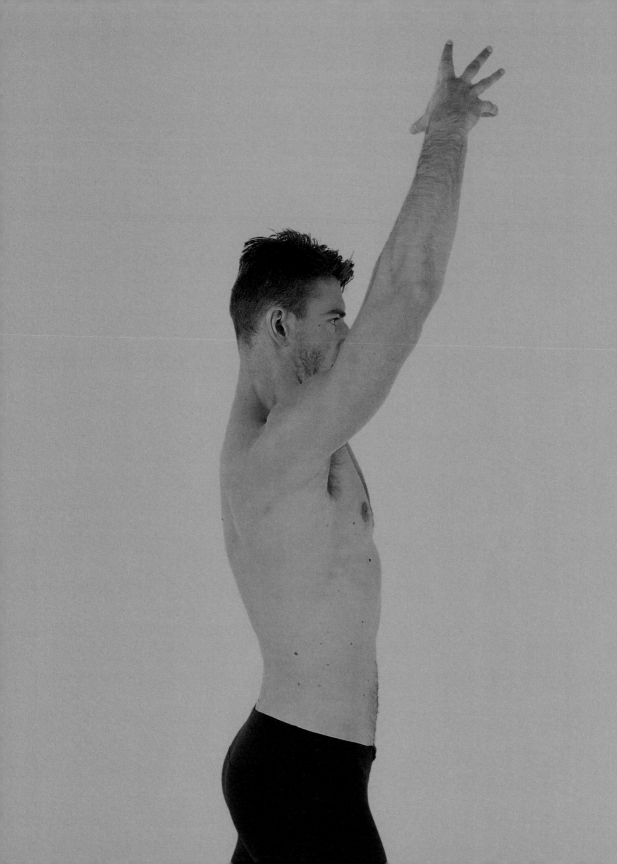

THREE

DECOMPRESS

Right now, please take three deep breaths, and as you breathe, notice how you're doing it. What's the process, and where is the air flowing? Hold on to your observations for now because this chapter is all about breathing, and by the end of the chapter, I suspect you may be breathing differently.

The chapter is about breathing because it is the essence of decompression and therefore is also the crucial element in these decompression exercises. A body compressed and grown rigid under gravity's excessive pressure is a body in which proper respiration has been stunted, effectively reining in every move the body makes and every stand it takes. Only lungs that are inflated to their oxygen-holding capacity are capable of empowering the appendicular skeleton to do everything it is capable of doing, and only a ribcage as big and wide as it can get can ensure that kind of lung power. These exercises are aimed therefore at reeducating the axial skeleton into an expansiveness that enables accurate, effective breathing—in effect, retraining the pulley systems around the ribcage to give that structure its maximum mechanical advantage, making it as big and wide as it can be so that the lungs can do their job successfully. It's as simple as that.

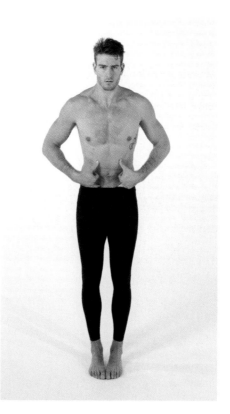

Forward-tilted head posture makes the ribcage and sternum weigh heavily on every breath you breathe.

But of course, the exercises constitute a change to the movement patterns and postural habits the body has fallen into—and that makes approaching these exercises not entirely simple. In some cases, the change may be radical, and in pretty much all cases, making the change won't be easy.

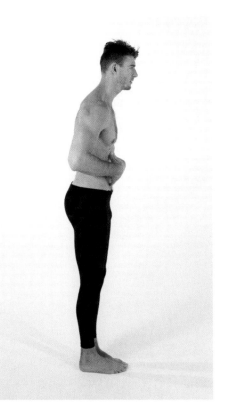

Forward-tilted head posture (profile view). Notice that his nose and toes are equal distance in front of his chest. Decompression breathing remedies this chronic position.

It's understandable. Years of defaulting to a "natural" posture that in fact was squeezed and constricted by gravity prompted the body to respond, out of sheer self-protection, into rigidity. Decompression movements confront that rigidity directly, and it requires no small effort to loosen things up.

So it is important to understand where that effort must come from—that is, the muscle work and the exertions of strength and energy that these decompression exercises are aimed at. What does this retraining of the axial skeleton require of the body, and what are the expected outcomes of the strengthening process? Three areas in particular are the focus of retraining in these decompression exercises: positioning the head, breathing with the diaphragm, and keeping the abdomen long and tight.

THE POSITION OF THE HEAD: SPACE AT THE BACK OF THE SKULL

In the decompression breathing at the heart of all the exercises in this chapter, the head needs to be positioned in such a way that the back of the skull, the occiput, is lifted off the neck. To visualize what that means, think of the skull and the tailbone pulling away from each other as far as they can, and position the head to make that distance happen.

One reason for positioning the head in this way, already observed

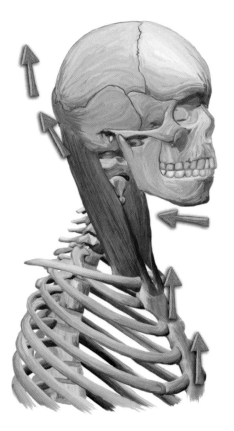

The base of the back of your skull must be pulled upward away from the backside bony protuberances of the cervical spine in order for the sternocleidomastoid muscle to optimally function.

in Hallie's case, is the central nervous system, significant branches of which travel from the brain through the occiput down the brain stem to the base of the spine, communicating along the way with the rest of the body. That won't happen as efficiently or as well as it should if the back of the skull rests on the neck and thereby denies space to that initial neural pathway through the occiput to the brain stem.

Equally significant is that when the occiput falls onto the neck, the angle of the shoulders shifts, causing the shoulders to droop downward. Yes, the shoulders belong to the appendicular skeleton, but they rest on the axial skeleton, and the jutting-forward head, positioned as in that bust of Queen Nefertiti, diminishes the support the axial skeleton can provide to hold the shoulders in place. So they droop, and the drooping shoulders in turn squeeze the ribcage and clavicles, and the muscle known as the pectoralis minor, which controls the angle of the shoulder blades, responds by shortening. When the pec minors get too short, they wrap the shoulders forward like a cloak over the clavicles and the ribcage—the rounded shoulders that are so common in so many of us. Conventional wisdom has long held that tight pec minor muscles pull the shoulder down, but it actually works the other way: Drooping shoulders contract the pec minor. Over time, shoulder droop accustoms the pec minors to the shortness—with often dire results, including numbness and tingling in the hands, a diminished pulse when the arms are lifted over the head, weakness in the upper body, even trouble in the jaw, because a jutting-forward head must constantly look up to find the horizon, and that affects the angle of the jaw.

Positioning the head to allow space at the base of the skull, by drawing a long line distancing the skull away from the pubic symphysis, resists and counters all that. The desired image is not the Queen Nefertiti profile but that of a prim, well-bred debutante forced to balance a book on her head. It may be a throwback to what was in many ways a restrictive era, but it can liberate, lengthen, and strengthen the axial skeleton in ways the shoulders, the ribcage, and your breathing will appreciate.

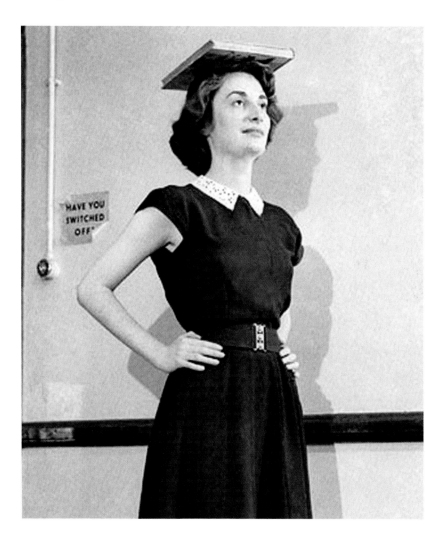

BREATHING WITH THE DIAPHRAGM

The second target of these exercises—one specifically addressing the respiratory process itself—is the need to fill out the ribcage as expansively as possible by pulling it away from center. The diaphragm initiates the expansion of the breathing process, contracting to enlarge the ribcage and thus increase the volume of the thoracic cavity, the great chamber of the body containing the heart and lungs, so that air can be drawn into the lungs during inhalation. What the decompression exercises of this chapter focus on is emphatically pulling the ribcage away from center so as to fill it completely, making certain in particular that air is funneled into the lower portion of the ribcage at the back, where compressed breathing rarely reaches.

Then comes exhalation, when the diaphragm relaxes. But in a body compressed by gravity, the muscle supporting that relaxing action, the serratus posterior, tends simply to collapse. Relaxation of the diaphragm is necessary, and it is the job of the serratus to enable it, but compression has swung the pendulum too far in the direction of relaxation—all the way to slump. The decompression exercises in this chapter are aimed at bringing the pendulum back into balance by retraining the serratus to maintain the expansion of the ribcage for a longer time in support of a more muscular exhalation.

Now think of the process as a whole, of your body pulling air into every corner of the ribcage so that it expands to the fullest extent possible on the inhale, then of letting the air out in gradual increments from the top of the ribcage to the bottom, so that the expansion is

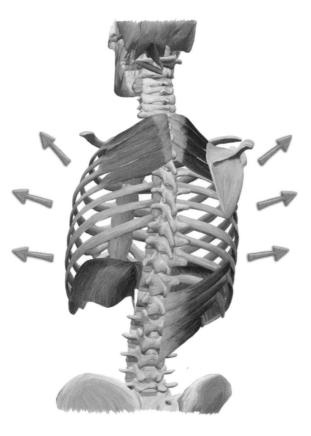

The diaphragm responds to the perimeter of the ribcage expanding outward away from its center. This uniform outward expansion is as primal as it gets when it comes to metabolically active muscular motions.

maintained to the very end of the exhale. That requires holding on to the contraction of the serratus for longer than a compressed serratus is accustomed to; it thus represents a significant change of habit for that muscle's action.

The contention that this change—which effectively makes the rib-cage work more muscularly—also makes for a more effective process of respiration and a more stable physical structure for the body has yet to be conclusively confirmed by research. It is time for such research to go forward and to analyze in depth what experience indicates—that a more expansive ribcage enabling greater lung inflation is a boon to the body's structure and well-being.

LENGTH IN THE ABDOMEN: A LONG, TIGHT CYLINDER

Finally, these decompression exercises focus on strengthening the ab-domen by lengthening it into a cylinder that is equally long and pow-erful all around, in every dimension. We know that a compressed and therefore shortened abdomen shifts the body's center of gravity, short-ening the spine and changing the biomechanics between the spine and the hip joint. Simply put, the shortened spine takes on the job the hip joint is supposed to do—namely, absorb the pressure of gravity. That makes for less effective muscle contraction throughout the body; it also typically makes for pain. A shortened spine causes the hip joints to rotate externally; they more or less spin the appendicular skeleton away from the axial skeleton, making space for the axial skeleton to collapse into—and thereby compress and shorten—the abdomen.

The result may feel like a tight abdomen; it can even take on the proverbial six-pack or washboard appearance. But its tightness is deceptive, an overcompensation that is a response to misuse. Tight as it may look or feel, that shortened, weakened abdomen actually prevents the body from using the muscles at the hip joint that maintain the center of gravity.

Lengthening the abdomen back to its true purpose and strength begins with decompression breathing. There are many different schools of thought on how best to brace the abdomen and muscularly support the important visceral tissue just beneath the abdominal muscle fibers; any and all of them will succeed better when the starting point is an abdomen lengthened by the decompression breathing of the exercises that follow.

DECOMPRESSION EXERCISES: READY, SET . . .

Ideally, the exercises should be performed in comfortable clothes and in bare feet on a bare floor or outside on a smooth plot of ground; in either location, you need enough room to stand or lie flat with your legs planted more than shoulder-width apart, plus sufficient space to extend your arms up and out and to be able to take a couple of steps both forward and back.

As for the number of repetitions you should do and the time it takes to go through this sequence of exercises, begin with the minimum defined for each exercise. As you grow more comfortable with the movements, it will be easy to add repetitions or spend more time.

What is crucial is to get the movements *right*. Results depend not on how forcefully or fervently these exercises are performed but on how well you support the body structurally and how frequently you move muscularly. Neurological re-patterning responds best to frequent small doses.

DECOMPRESSION BREATHING

The decompression breath is the core of these exercises. In fact, each of the exercises that follow the description of decompression breathing is simply a different posture in which to perform the decompression breath.

Obviously, the process of respiration—passing oxygen into the bloodstream and removing carbon dioxide from it—is the essential physiological task of life. Compressed lungs cheat that essential physiological task; they don't do it well enough or completely enough. Decompression breathing corrects that. It is estimated that the body takes anywhere from 23,000 to 25,000 breaths each day, so even a handful of breaths done right will decrease the carbon dioxide in the lungs by enough to leave more room for oxygen and make the body feel and perform better.

In fact, a small note of caution is in order: In my experience, about one in ten people feel a bit light-headed the very first time they try a real decompression breath and expand their ribcage to its fullest. They don't faint, and the light-headedness occurs only the very first time they do the breath, but there's a chance it may happen to you. My theory is that in the people who do experience this slightly woozy sensation, the lung's alveolar sacs are expelling the residue of carbon dioxide that has lingered there for who knows how long. The cure is a few more decompression breaths to purge it entirely.

In doing a decompression breath, it helps to visualize your lungs inside your ribcage: a pair of bellows-like sacs ready to be filled to the maximum with the air you bring to them. The cage that protects them—the ribs are the slats of the cage—is oblong in shape and rounded, and the higher it can be lifted and the wider its roundness can be expanded, the better the chance of achieving maximum inflation of the lungs. Keep that in mind as you begin your decompression breathing.

Start by making sure your head is lifted off the neck and is positioned for space at the back of the skull. To make it happen, mentally stretch a long line from your skull to your tailbone, holding your chin in and elongating your neck. For a helpful tool, use a Shaka sign on both hands. Place your thumbs on the lowest rib you can feel on the ribcage and place your pinky finger on the upper rim of your pelvis. The space between pinky and thumb should increase with every breath in Foundation Training.

Inhale. Don't shrug or hike up your shoulders; instead, raise your sternum, letting the breath of the inhalation lift your ribcage upward

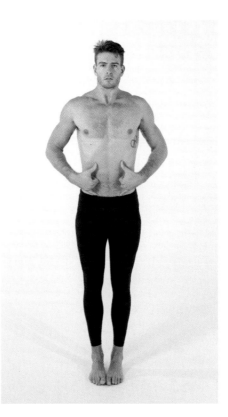

Place your thumbs at the bottom of your ribcage. Place your small finger at the top of your pelvis (called the anterior superior iliac spine). Use this as a measuring stick for basic decompression breathing. Each inhale should increase the space between fingers. Each exhale is meant to maintain that space.

from the hips as you press your abdomen in toward the navel. Bring the air into your lung as your ribcage expands evenly front, back, and sides—all around, not neglecting the lower back portion of the ribcage. You want your ribcage to ride up on the air you're breathing into it and to open up fully. You want to feel it mounting from below—ascending on the inhalation, not being hauled up from above—as the lungs fill.

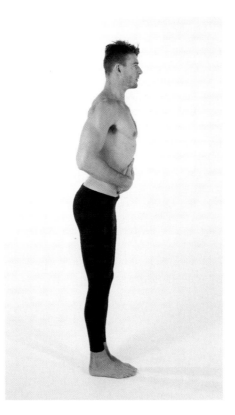

Keep your chin back as your sternum (the center of your chest) lifts up. My favorite cue is "Chin back, chest up." Let your hips support you by hinging them back slightly.

Exhale. Pull your abdomen in tight and maintain the expansion and elevation of the ribcage as long as you can as you let the breath out. Hold on to the tension in all those muscles you've elongated during the inhalation and let the lungs deflate step by step, from the top of the ribcage to the bottom.

The minimum for doing the decompression breath is three repetitions. Do the decompression breath whenever you can, but certainly do it three times or more in succession in the morning on awakening, three times or more in the afternoon, three times or more before bed, and during every Foundation Training exercise.

To me there's a kind of magic in decompression breathing, although it's a pretty straightforward matter of biomechanical science. Standing tall against gravity by expanding the ribcage and filling your lungs with air is the gateway to everything else in the body's natural posture of strength and flexibility. When the ribcage is as big as it can be all the way around, chances are good that you're long and strong in the torso, with an axial skeleton elongated from the tailbone to the skull. Everything is supported.

THE SEVEN DECOMPRESSION EXERCISES

The remaining exercises in the chapter take this decompression breathing into seven separate postures that pit your body against gravity in seven different ways, as well as into one corrective challenge to the shoulders, which the axial skeleton supports. Two of the gravity-confronting postures do it straight up and head-on, two of them at a 90-degree angle to the force of gravity from the earth's plane—on your back to strengthen the front of your body, on your front to strengthen the back of your body. A fifth posture challenges gravity while you are kneeling, and the sixth with your body seated, perhaps the most common and unfortunately the most unhealthful circumstance of contemporary life. Each of these postures also helps expand the space within the torso, making more room for the tissue and organs that keep us functioning.

The seventh exercise, called shoulder tracing, challenges the breakdown of full rotation in the shoulder and strengthens the muscles affected by that breakdown. Shoulders that don't rotate as they should become rounded and rigid; they fall, compressing the axial skeleton that supports them. That's why, although shoulders are part of the appendicular skeleton, the shoulder tracing exercise affects decompression in general.

1. STANDING DECOMPRESSION

The standing decompression posture is a direct challenge to the force of gravity.

Stand with your feet parallel—big toes touching one another and heels separated by one to two inches—and with your weight on your heels. Keep your arms at your sides, elbows slightly bent, palms forward, and with your thumbs externally rotated so that your chest and shoulders are open.

Make sure your feet are planted firmly on the floor—or on the ground if you are outside, of course—and that your weight is on your heels. From this planted position, the aim is to make yourself tall through breathing.

Begin by inhaling a decompression breath, raising and broadening your ribcage as expansively as possible, keeping the head positioned for space at the back of the skull, holding the chin in and the neck long. Maintain the expansion as you exhale, pressing your abdomen in toward your navel.

Try to get taller with each repetition.

Each full decompression breath, combining inhale and exhale should take 10 to 15 seconds.

MINIMUM: three repetitions, one per minute

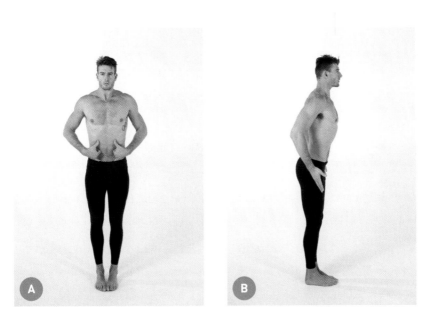

A. Stand tall with the ball of the big toes touching each other and the heels 1 inch apart to line up your pelvis.

B. Open the arms with the elbows slightly bent. Use the upper back and mid-back muscles to expand your chest. Thumbs point away from each other.

C. Lift the arms without straining your neck. Push the crown of your head back and up as the arms lift. Expand the torso and press the ball of the big toe into the ground.

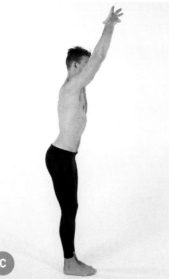

2. LUNGE DECOMPRESSION

It's easy to go right into the lunge decompression from the standing decompression position, and it's an exercise that lets you almost feel your abdomen lengthening as you do it.

Step forward on the right leg and step the left leg back; you are now in a standing lunge. The distance of the lunge is immaterial— short or long—so long as both feet face straight ahead and your hips are squared. The front foot should be flat on the floor, while the heel of your back foot should be raised, toes gripping the floor.

Raise both arms straight up high over your head and touch fingertips. Press your feet into the floor. Do a decompression breath for 30 seconds while holding your stance. Then do two more 30-second breaths. With every inhalation, expand your ribcage more expansively and try to stand taller—that is, taller and more expansive on the second breath than on the first, taller and more expansive than that on the third breath. Remain tall and maintain the expansion on the exhale.

After three breaths, lower your arms, and from a normal standing position, reverse the position of the standing lunge—left leg in front, right leg back, hips squared, front foot flat on the floor, back foot with heel raised. Again, lift your arms straight up to the ceiling joining hands at the fingertips as you take three decompression breaths, each one taller and with a more expansive ribcage than the one before. At this point, in fact, your abdomen is likely to be tightening a bit each time you raise your torso.

MINIMUM: three repetitions; one repetition = 30 seconds, three breaths on each leg

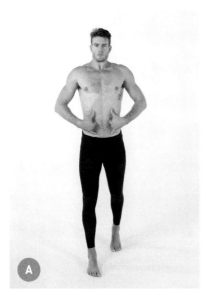

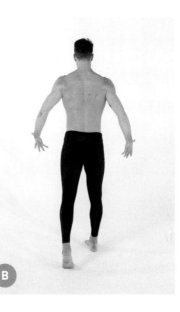

Stand tall with the ball of the big toes touching each other and the heels 1 inch apart to line up your pelvis.

A. Stand tall with one leg in front of the other in a strong and tall split stance. Keep your hips square.

B. Open the arms with the elbows slightly bent. Use the upper back and mid-back muscles to expand your chest. Thumbs point away from each other.

C. Lift the arms without straining your neck. As the arms lift, try to squeeze the inner thighs toward each other like a weak pair of scissors.

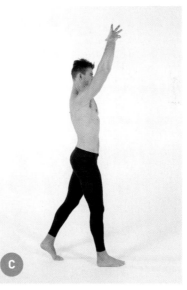

3. SUPINE DECOMPRESSION

In effect, you'll now take the standing decompression position onto your back. Perpendicular to the force of gravity but offering a wider area for dispersal of the force, the supine position enables emphasis on the muscles in the front of the body that support the elongation of the torso and the expansion of your ribcage in decompression breathing.

Lie on your back, feet parallel and touching, with the tops of the feet flexed and pulled toward the shins. Bend your knees just enough to be able to squeeze your inner thighs together. Begin the decompression breath, lengthening your torso away from your hips as you expand your ribcage and as your sternum rises on the breath. Maintain the expansion as you exhale.

MINIMUM: three repetitions

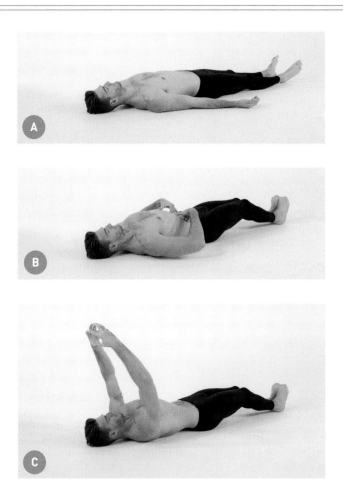

A. Begin in a relaxed supine pose and then bring the feet and knees together.

B. There should be a subtle bend in your knees, which will help you rotate the hips and thighs toward each other until the groin muscles begin to fatigue. Hold that position.

C. Squeeze the upper inner thighs without squeezing your butt muscles. Lift the arms above the chest without straining your neck. Deep breaths will expand your ribcage posteriorly toward the ground.

4. PRONE DECOMPRESSION

This is the companion-piece to supine decompression; it further strengthens the front of the body from the most expansive position the body can assume.

Lie on your front, feet parallel and touching, with your toes tucked and curled under, giving the arch a good stretch. Again squeeze the knees and inner thighs together. With your arms out in front of you, press your fingertips into the ground or floor and lift your forehead and nose off the ground as you elevate your chest, making sure to position your head for space at the base of the skull.

Breathe. Expand the ribcage and lengthen it away from the hips as you inhale, and maintain the expansion as you exhale, keeping the abdomen tight. Do the decompression breath four times, and with each breath, stretch and press a little more: Press the fingertips into the floor and squeeze the knees harder; position the head with chin pulled back and neck lengthened even further; stretch the feet a little longer. Four breaths constitute one repetition.

MINIMUM: three repetitions; one repetition = four decompression breaths

---

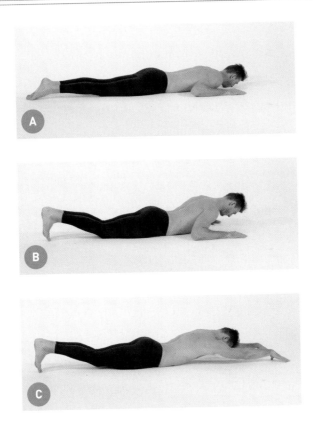

A. Begin in a prone position and bring your feet and legs together. Your toes and knees should remain on the ground for the entire prone decompression exercise.

B. Pull your chin and nose straight away from the floor, do not extend your neck to look upward. Make your neck long and keep your chin back. Reach your arms forward.

C. With the arms forward, as wide as they must be for comfort, press the fingertips to the ground and pull the wrists and elbows away from the ground. Your abdomen, neck, chest, arm, and shoulder muscles should begin to fatigue. This is not a cobra pose or a Superman-type back extension. This pose is meant to lengthen the spine, not to extend it.

5. KNEELING DECOMPRESSION

Bring your body to a kneeling position. Maintain weight through your knees with a pad or rolled-up mat between your kneecaps and the floor. Your knees should be hip-width apart. Position yourself as tall as possible with your feet directly behind you. Point your heels toward the sky by contracting your shin muscles.

Make sure that all of your body weight is over your knees, not on the feet; if the weight goes through your feet you will be contracting your abdomen and hip flexors harder than your posterior chain muscles, and you want the posterior chain to hold you up while kneeling. Instead, keep the weight on the knees, take a deep decompression breath, and slowly hinge your hips back until you feel the muscles of the back and hips supporting the weight of your torso.

This exercise is great for people who have trouble with some of our standing exercises; it can also be among the biggest challenges for larger people who have forgotten how to hinge their hips well.

This position should feel like you are about to fall forward, but the posterior chain muscles will stop that fall when the exercise is practiced well.

MINIMUM: **three repetitions of three breaths**

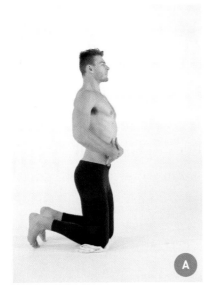

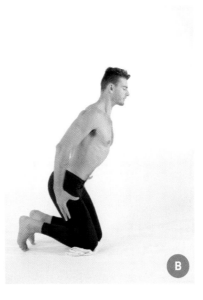

A. Kneel on a mat or towel. Keep your weight through the knees and lightly touch the floor with your toes. If the toes come off the ground, try to remain balanced. Chin back, chest up. If this position still hurts, avoid it.

B. Counterbalance your weight by hinging the hips back and lifting the torso up and forward. Keep the weight through your knees. Keep your feet light.

C. Reach the arms forward as you pull the hips back to add even more resistance to the hip hinge. Stay strong and expand your torso with decompression breaths.

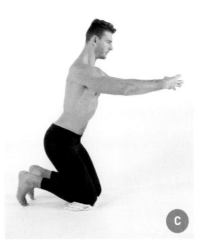

6. SEATED DECOMPRESSION

This is of course the toughest of the decompression breathing postures. You may even sweat a bit as you work your way through the
repetitions; in fact, you probably should work at it hard enough to
raise a bit of a glow.

If the seat you use for the exercise is adjustable, by all means set
the seatback as a tool to align your torso straight up.

Without such a tool, sit forward on the seat, away from the backrest,
as tall as you can with your weight directly on your sit bones. Extend
your legs if you can, but keep your heels on the floor and pull your toes
back toward your shins. Squeeze your knees together. If possible, use
a prop that makes this action more effective: a water bottle, rolled-up
sweater, book, even a wad of paper placed between the knees.

Position your head for space at the back of the skull—chin drawn
in, neck long. Place your hands on either side of your body, ready to
measure between little finger and thumb the distance, when you are
at the top of the breath inhalation, between the top of your pelvis and
the bottom of your ribcage. Begin the decompression breath, expanding the ribcage and elongating the torso as your sternum rises on the
breath. Measure the top-of-pelvis to bottom-of-ribcage distance on both
hands, then begin your exhalation. Brace your abdomen; try to maintain the same measured distance on the exhale that you achieved with
the inhale. And of course, with each repetition, try for more expansiveness, higher lift, and tighter control of the abdomen on the exhale.

MINIMUM: three breaths

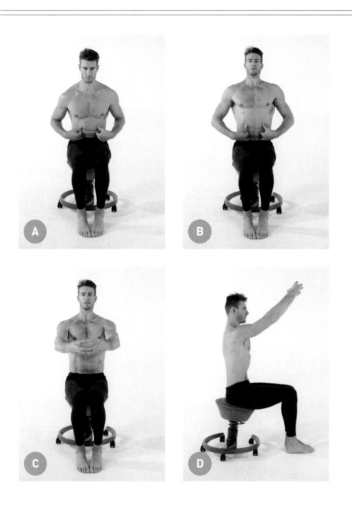

A. Slide toward the end of your chair and sit as tall as you can.

B. Bring the ankles directly under the front of your knees and squeeze your feet and knees together.

C. Sit as tall as you can, squeeze your knees, and take 3 forceful decompression breaths.

D. Bring the arms up at chest height into a Sphere of Tension. Take another 3 to 5 decompression breaths and repeat as needed.

7. SHOULDER TRACING

In this exercise, you trace the path of your shoulder's natural rotation, and in so doing, you begin to correct the breakdown that has occurred in the joint through too much internal rotation. That rotation has shortened the muscles that support the shoulder—specifically, the pectoral muscles and the sternocleidomastoid, the thick neck muscle at the top of the shoulder that actually starts in the sternum and clavicle. Shoulder tracing challenges those muscles, forcing the shoulder to move against them by seamlessly coursing through the full range of motion the shoulder joint is capable of. Because the shoulders are a weight above the torso, they need to be repositioned if the axial skeleton is to expand properly; that's why this movement is so important to decompression.

The movement is done by the thumbs with the elbows extended as levers. There's nothing forced or forceful about shoulder tracing, although paradoxically it will help to undo any number of shoulder impairments. The key is to practice decompression breathing throughout the movement.

Stand with feet apart, arms at your sides with palms facing backward and your elbows bent so that your thumbs are touching the exact midpoint of each side. Hinge back at the hip.

Use your thumbs as pointers to trace each side of your body upward as your elbows bend increasingly outward from your sides and away from one another. Be sure to keep your arms in the same plane as your torso, neither ahead of it nor behind it, and keep the wrists straight.

When your thumbs reach your armpits, stop tracing with the

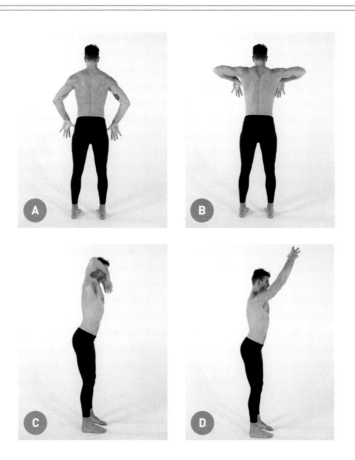

A. Stand tall with the thumbs pressing into your greater trochanter, the bony spot on the side of your hips. It is lower than you think!

B. Keep your elbows as wide as possible and your neck relaxed as you slowly lift the arms to trace the thumbs up the flank of your body.

C. Elbows stay up as high as possible. Do not flex your wrists to get up higher; it is the elbow joint that lifts the arms up higher and higher. Chin back, chest up.

D. Once the elbows are as high as they can go, slowly bring the hands up the back of the head until they can reach up and forward as tall as they can be. Again, do not strain your neck to do this.

thumbs but keep raising your elbows up, up, up toward the sky and diagonally away from your sternum, so that the backs of your hands are near the sides of your face.

Externally rotate the shoulders till your hands are behind your neck. Keep your head and neck drawn back and the nape of the neck long.

Straighten your arms as you extend them overhead and bring your fingertips together in a Sphere of Tension.

Shoulder tracing is a remarkable facilitator for greater range of motion in this naturally powerful joint and is therefore the perfect wrap-up for decompressing your spine through these postures and movements.

MINIMUM: **three repetitions**

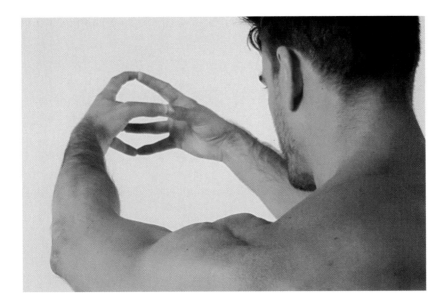

To hold a powerful Sphere of Tension, imagine your hand holding a balloon that is fully expanded and you can just barely reach around the whole thing. Then press the hands together in that position. All of the joints in the fingers are unlocked and the hands press together with 5 to 10 pounds of pressure.

Take three deep breaths again. I'll wager the process feels completely different now, and so it should. You now know how and why breathing happens inside the lungs, which need space, protected within an expansible ribcage, to function well. That is why an expansive axial skeleton is the essential foundation for a decompressed body that can resist gravity naturally.

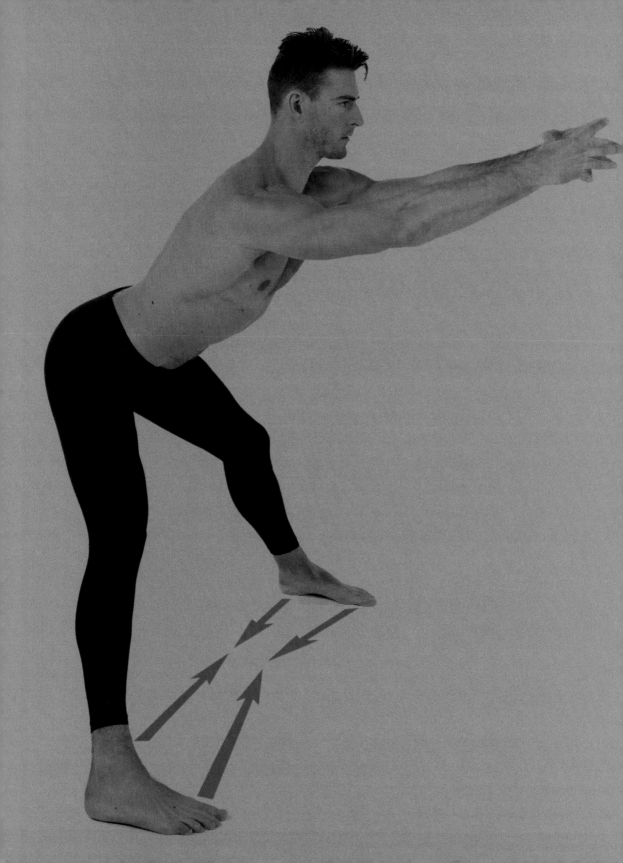

FOUR

GET ANCHORED

Think of the pelvis as the platform from which the axial skeleton pulls upward and outward. An equal downward and outward pull from the bottom of the pelvic platform is essential for maintaining the tension that supports the entire structure, and that is precisely what the appendicular skeleton supplies. From the pelvis down to the toes, the anchoring power of the appendicular skeleton gives the axial skeleton something stable to pull against. It rounds out the job of keeping the body's frame expansive.

This chapter provides exercises that strengthen and lengthen the muscles that do that anchoring. They are the muscles that attach the lower limbs of the appendicular skeleton to the pelvic platform—in particular, the gluteal, hamstring, iliacus, and adductor muscles. These are the muscles that hold us upright and, as the movers of the hip joint, propel us—via rotation, extension, and flexion—in all sorts of directions through various planes and axes. They are at their optimum mechanical advantage when they pull the base of the pelvis

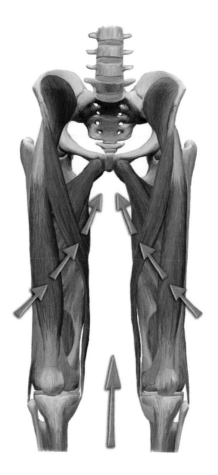

Anchoring muscles are designed to provide healthy opposition to the muscles of the outer hips, like the glutes. If you have chronically tight glutes and hamstrings, fix them long term by strengthening these anchoring muscles.

and the thighbone toward one another, and that is precisely what the exercises in this chapter aim for.

There are four exercises. To ensure that all are done from as close to that optimum mechanical advantage as possible, start with internal leg tracing. Just as shoulder tracing, in the previous chapter, challenged the breakdown of the shoulder's external rotation, internal leg tracing challenges the breakdown of the hips' internal rotation, tightening the muscles on the inside of the leg in order to produce the natural reciprocal reaction to that, which is for the muscles along the outside of the hips to lengthen and strengthen. This primes the whole appendicular skeleton for the anchoring exercises that follow and positions the body for squeezing full effectiveness from each of the exercises you do.

Something else that gets strengthened in these anchoring exercises is the feet. Today's lifestyles offer us little opportunity for strengthening our feet, which, understandably, we spend a lot of time and money protecting from the surfaces they walk on. The result, however, is that our feet tend to lack gripping power and flexibility; we more or less slap them onto the ground as if they were just useless appendages, which they are in danger of becoming. In fact, however, the foot muscles are key in anchoring the body in our aboveground sea of gravity. Toes can and should grip as they curl and flex; the muscles of the arch store energy, act as springs, and protect us from musculoskeletal damage; the muscles of the sole move the toes and support the arch and deserve to be planted firmly. So putting your feet to work is essential in helping you push back against gravity. Use them to grab hold of the earth or to grip the floor you're standing on. Stretch and flex and move your toes. Stand as firmly and as solidly as you stand big and tall, as you anchor your skeletal structure into whatever surface you're standing on.

1. INTERNAL LEG TRACING

Again, this is the kickoff exercise that sets the tone for the anchoring exercises to follow. What shoulder tracing did by challenging the adapted internal rotation of shoulder breakdown, internal leg tracing does by challenging the adapted external rotation of the hips and anchoring the inner leg muscles.

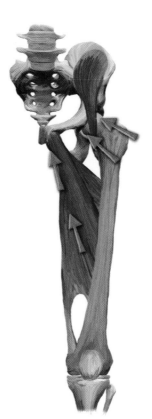

The iliacus and adductor muscles are among the many muscles that pull the head of the femur deeply into its joint socket, the acetabulum. This maneuver facilitates the varied circumduction motions of the leg.

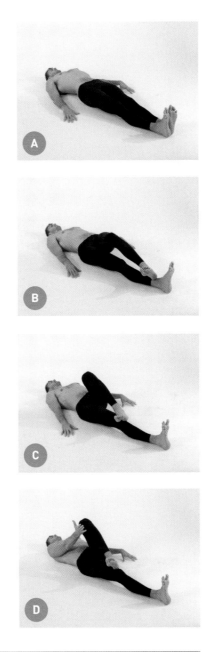

A. Begin in a supine position much like a supine decompression.

B. Lift one leg, internally rotate it from the hip to the big toe and then place that heel on top of the opposite shin.

C. Trace the heel of the top leg all the way up the shin until you reach the kneecap or slightly above the kneecap. Maintain internal rotation.

D. Press the palm of the opposite hand against the inside of the knee. Ten pounds of pressure should do the trick. The anchoring muscles along the inner leg should begin to fatigue. Maintain the same steady internal rotation as you trace the heel all the way back down the shin and repeat on the other side.

Too much sitting, a fact of life for just about every single one of us, shortens the gluteal muscles that are necessary to support proper hip rotation, so this tracing focuses on the iliacus and the adductor, the muscles on the inside of the thigh that "oppose" the gluteals. As iliacus and adductor are strengthened, they become capable of resisting the muscles on the back of the leg that keep trying to rotate externally. As one limb traces another and unnaturally shortened muscles are lengthened, the body learns to return to its natural symmetry, and the rotational capability can again work through the full range of motion that is its natural state.

Here's how:

Lie on your back, arms at your sides, palms down. Feet are dorsiflexed—that is, bent dorsally, toward their upper surface. Curl your toes and point your feet together till the big toes are touching as you bend your knees up, raising them slightly off the floor.

With the feet still dorsiflexed and the toes still tightly curled, lift your right leg, bend it to the left, and lay your right heel on the top surface of your left foot so that it is aimed across the midline of the body; it should maintain that aim through the tracing movement. Trace the left leg with the heel of the right foot up along the shin, the kneecap, and the first few inches of the lower thigh—no farther. When your bent right knee is at a 90-degree angle to the plane of your body, raise your left arm and place the left palm against the right knee. Push the palm and the knee against one another and hold for 10 seconds.

Raise both arms straight up, fingertips of the two hands tented and touching, and pull your arms back till they are over your face.

Hold this position for 5 seconds, then lower your arms to your sides, palms down on the floor.

Trace your right heel down the left leg till both feet, still dorsiflexed with toes curled, are together and touching.

Lift the left leg, bend the left foot rightward, and set the left heel on the top surface of the right foot aimed across the midline of the body. Trace up the right leg with the left heel. When the left knee forms a 90-degree angle with the plane of the body, raise your right hand and push the palm against the knee in mutual resistance. Hold for 10 seconds.

Reach both arms, with tented hands touching at the fingertips, back and over the face, hold, then return arms to your sides. Left leg retraces down the right leg till both feet, still dorsiflexed with toes curled, are together and touching.

Uncurl the toes and let the feet separate and the body return to neutral.

The focus throughout the entire movement is to internally rotate both legs, particularly the thighbone.

You're now ready to get anchored and to take that anchoring stance into two key postures.

2. GETTING ANCHORED

Start on your feet. They should be a comfortable distance apart—
about hip-width from one another—but with the outside lines of the
feet parallel. Unlock your knees, and shift your weight onto your heels.
Now lift the toes of both feet simultaneously. Spread the toes out as
wide as you can, then lower them back to the floor.

What you're doing in this process is supporting your legs from
the inside of the thighs to the arches. To get it right, you'll need to
convince yourself that your arches are being pulled upward away from
the ground, not simply lifting up. It is the fascia of your body that is
pulling the arch up—that all-encompassing, weblike fabric of tissue
that holds your body together. It draws the arch up toward your groin,
pulling also a whole network of small connecting muscles, and it feels
like you are squeezing your legs toward each other without the knees
moving inward.

The succeeding anchoring exercises in this chapter all need to be
done in this anchored way, with legs together to strengthen the muscles from arches to thighs, and making sure the knees don't cave in.

MINIMUM: one repetition three times a day

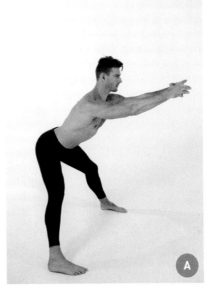

A. Assume a wide stance hinging at the hips.

B. To this position, add a somewhat symmetrical inward pull. It is not the only way to significantly improve your muscular recruitment, but it is one of the most effective methods. Keep your feet, knees, and ankles strong as you pull inward from the hips, heels, and toes.

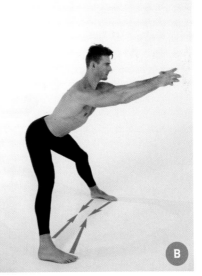

3. ANCHORED BRIDGE

Here's a way to activate your posterior chain as you lengthen the hamstrings that are key to the appendicular skeleton's downward pull. Lie down on your back, with your big toes touching so that your outside arches are parallel. Pull the tops of your feet back toward your shins as you bend the knees just enough for your inner thighs to touch. You should feel your thighbones rolling inward as you draw your inner thighs together.

Squeeze your inner thighs tighter as you bend your knees till they are anywhere from eight inches to a foot above the floor.

Press your heels and the backs of your arms into the floor or ground surface and pull your hips up. Keep your heels ground into the floor, the thighs tight together, and the back of your neck long as you practice decompression breathing in this posture.

MINIMUM: one repetition three times a day

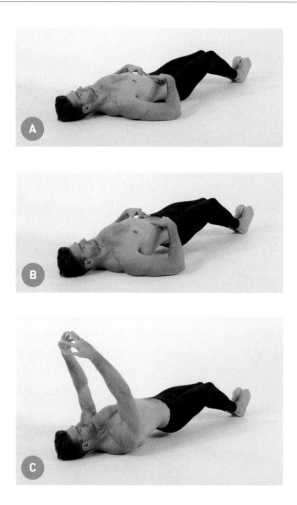

A. Begin supine with legs together and knees bent slightly so that they are not any higher than your chest.

B. Isometrically pull your heels toward your hips without moving them. It feels like the back of the legs activate quickly.

C. Continue pulling the heels toward the hips and squeeze your knees as you lift the hips 1 to 3 inches off the ground.

4. ANCHORED BACK EXTENSION

In this extension, your anchoring muscles sustain the grip that pulls the pelvis away from the ribcage. Lie on your front, feet parallel and touching with your toes curled under, head down so you're looking at the floor. Bend your elbows and hold them close to your sides with your hands under your shoulders.

Bend your knees just enough to lift your toes off the ground as you squeeze your inner thighs together and lift your arms, head, and chest up from the ground. Be sure to keep your elbows and hands in the same position as when you started: elbows close to your sides, hands under the shoulder. Pull your chin back and elongate the back of your neck as you inhale a decompression breath and maintain the lift on exhalation.

MINIMUM: one repetition three times a day

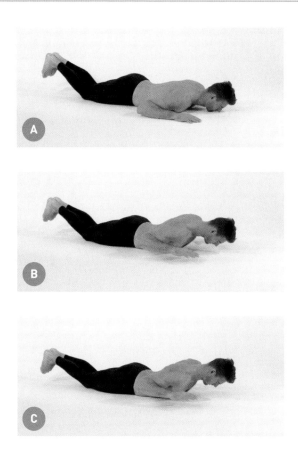

A. Begin prone with knees together and feet a few inches off the ground. The knees remain on the ground.

B. Pull the chin, chest, wrist, and elbows off the ground as you squeeze the knees a bit harder.

C. Take several decompression breaths trying to lengthen your torso with each inhalation. Maintain your height and expansion with each exhalation. Keep the knees together and tight.

Each of these anchoring exercises should be held for the length of from five to seven breaths, which should take from 30 to 60 seconds, and should be repeated three times a day. Along with the internal leg tracing that begins the sequence and primes the body for getting the most out of the exercises, the full complement of this anchoring "workout" amounts to perhaps 5 or 6 minutes, time easily carved out of even the busiest day.

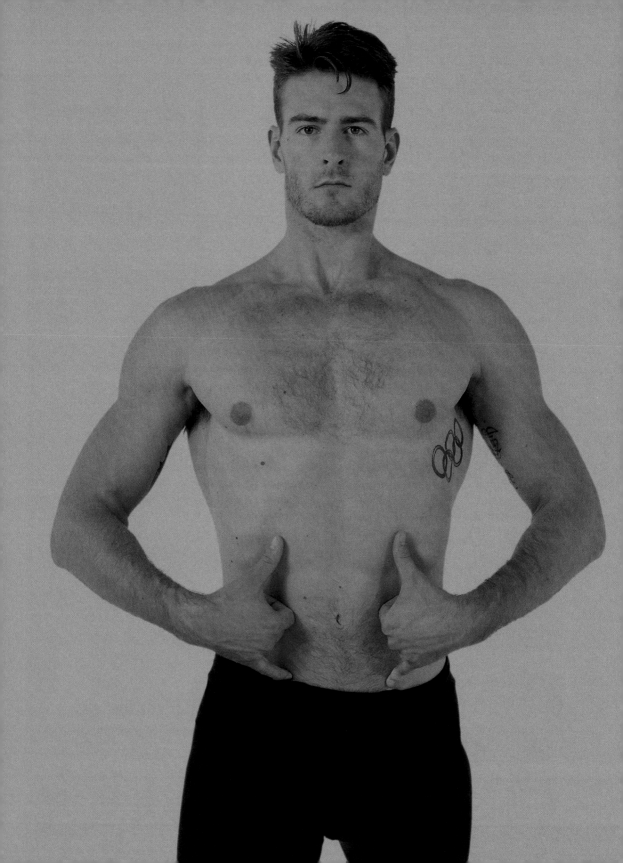

FIVE

THE WRAP-UP

QUARTET

The decompression and anchoring exercises of the previous two chapters are boot camp—basic training for restoring your body's natural physical foundation. In this chapter, a quartet of wrap-up exercises gives those basics a final flourish, integrating and affirming the training and tying it all together. I think of this wrap-up quartet as topping up the tug-of-war between axial and appendicular, giving the tension between the two an extra push for good measure. Spend time with the movements and postures of Chapters 3 and 4, but round out and reinforce what you're trying to accomplish with the four exercises of this wrap-up.

1. FOUNDER

The founder is absolutely basic to the entire Foundation Training toolkit. It is the granddaddy of postures—the primary recruiter of the posterior chain of muscles, the key to ensuring that the body hinges at the hip, and a core movement for decompression, and it is probably the best way I know of to put yourself on the fast track to spinal stability, hip mobility, and a body in better balance.

Stand with your feet facing forward as much as three feet apart, with the outside lines of the feet parallel to one another and your weight on your heels. Get anchored, lifting the toes of both feet, then lowering them to the floor. Stand tall, with your chest up and your sternum raised.

Unlock your hips, hinge them backward, and pull them out behind your heels, making sure your abdomen stays long. Knees bend slightly but stay well behind the toes.

As you feel tension in the lower back, unscrew the shoulders by opening the hands, separating the fingers wide, and turning the thumbs outward.

From this position, move your arms forward touching the hands together at the fingertips as you counterbalance the backward-hinging hip movement.

Start the tug of war: Reach forward with your arms, pull back with your hips—simultaneously—while keeping your chest high and your weight pressed into your heels.

Hold the posture as you breathe a high, wide, full decompression breath and maintain the expansion on the exhale.

Stand up.

MINIMUM: one repetition three times a day

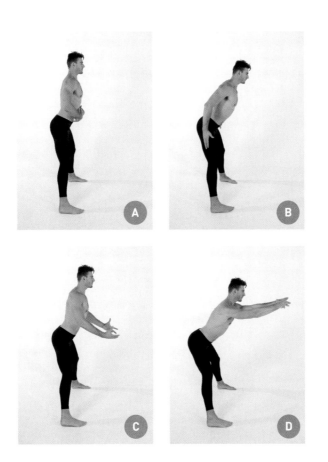

A. Begin in a wide stance with feet firmly pressing toward the ground, take 3 decompression breaths.

B. Open the arms, expand your chest, and hinge your hips back well behind your feet. Allow the knees to gently unlock. The knees must remain above or behind the ankles.

C. Scoop arms forward and up as you hinge the hips farther back.

D. Once you find a challenging counterbalance between the hips and arms, hold the pose for 3 to 5 more decompression breaths.

2. WOODPECKER

Woodpeckers—the avian kind, not the exercises—have what's called a zygodactyl foot, with two toes facing front and one facing back, so that they always appear forward-looking as they climb. The Foundation Training posture approximates the look by hinging at the hip and splitting the legs forward and back, lengthening the gluteal muscles supporting and propelling the back-pulling hip and adding leverage to the posterior chain.

Stand with your feet parallel and your hips square, arms open and turned out at your sides. Take a high, wide, full decompression inhalation and hinge at the hips with one leg stepping forward; then pull the hip back. The front foot is flat on the floor and the front knee is behind the ankle; the foot of the back leg is raised at the heel for the added leverage. Bring the arms forward for counterbalance, the hands touching at the fingertips.

Do several decompression breaths in this position, then return to a standing position: feet parallel and hips square, arms open and turned out at the sides. Breathe again and hinge at the hips, bringing the other leg forward, then pulling that hip back. With back heel raised and front knee behind the ankle, bring the arms forward and up for counterbalance, touching the hands at the fingertips. After several decompression breaths in this position, return to the standing position.

MINIMUM: one repetition three times

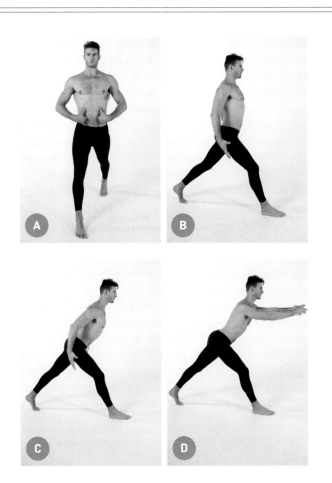

A. Step into a tall split stance with the hips squared and the front knee slightly bent. Take 3 decompression breaths.

B. Open the arms and chest as you hinge the hips back to load the posterior chain of your front leg.

C. Once you feel a stretch and fatigue in the hamstrings and low back, bring your arms forward to counterbalance deeper.

D. Keep the chin back and chest up for 3 to 5 more decompression breaths.

3. WOODPECKER ROTATION

This exercise adds a rotational move to the woodpecker posture in order to force the gluteal and adductor muscles actively to support the whole weight of the torso. The aim is to make the glutes the strongest part of the body, as they should be.

From the top of the posture—that is, hinged at the hip with one leg forward and its foot flat on the floor, knee behind the ankle, with the back foot raised at the heel, and with arms stretched out in front of you, fingertips touching—begin rotating your pelvis in the direction of the front leg. Keeping all of your weight on that leg, and with the front heel gripping the floor, let your torso and arms follow the pelvis in its rotation till the entire upper body has pivoted about ten inches and no more than twelve inches. Rotate back inward, maintaining the contraction in the gluteal muscles and the pressure in the front heel.

Do three rotations, then return to a standing position and begin the posture with the other leg forward.

MINIMUM: one repetition (three rotations) three times

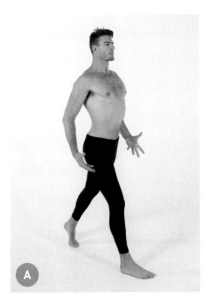

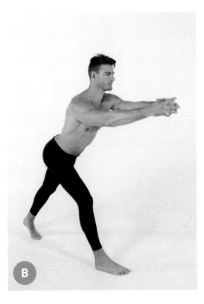

A. Step into a tall split stance with the hips squared and the front knee slightly bent. Take 3 decompression breaths.

B. Open the arms and chest as you hinge the hips back to load the posterior chain of your front leg.

C. Bring the arms forward, load all your weight to the front leg and rotate three to six inches to the same side as the front leg. This should make your glute muscles fatigue quickly.

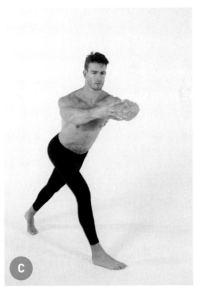

4. INTEGRATED HINGES

These graduated hinging movements remind the body that movement originates in the core and that the hip is not just the body's great shaker but also its main mover—and that the right movement is a hinge, especially, for example, when you are lifting something.

Stand with the feet shoulder-width apart and parallel, your weight on the heels and your toes gripping the floor.

Bend your elbows and hold them close to your sides with your hands in front of and just below the shoulders.

Decompress: Breathe high, wide, and fully and anchor the lower body, pressing your weight onto your heels, raising and spreading your toes, and tensing your inner thighs.

Unlock the knees, keep your weight in your heels, and without moving your spine, hinge slightly at the hip, pulling the hips back behind the heels.

Pull the hips farther and farther back, in stages.

Drive your weight into your heels and push against the floor as you lift your torso, also in stages, and return to a neutral position.

MINIMUM: one repetition three times a day

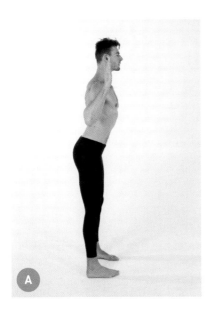

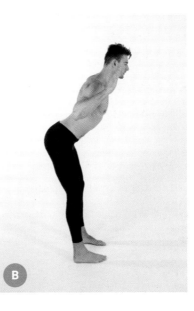

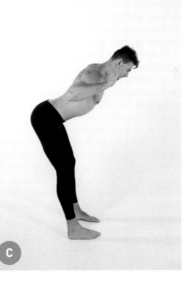

A. Stand tall with legs in any width position you choose—wide, narrow, hip width, shoulder width.

B. Bend your elbows to bring your hands by your ears. This is another chance to keep your chest wide and your back strong as you hinge.

C. Keep your spine long, still, and stable as your hips do all of the work to hinge you back and forth slowly. Try to perform 5 to 10 integrated hinges for each rep.

This wrap-up quartet of exercises provides the finishing touch only to a sequence of exercises that need to be repeated frequently. It cannot be stressed too often or too strongly that restoring your body's natural strength and flexibility comes not through intensity of effort but through consistency. The body responds to how well and how persistently the postures and movements of Foundation Training are performed, not to how hard you do them. As the next chapter details, the aim is to make these postures and movements your normal way of holding yourself structurally and moving muscularly.

PART THREE

Sustained Pain Relief and Everyday Fitness

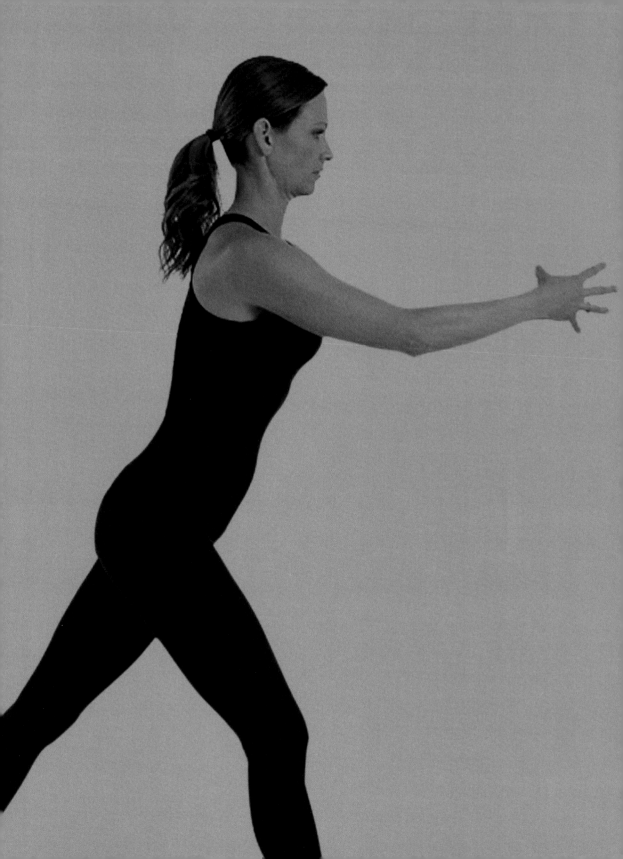

SIX

DAY BY DAY

They say you can't really claim fluency in a foreign language until you've dreamed in the language—in other words, until it's lodged in your subconscious.

The metaphor works for Foundation Training as well: You can only claim that your body is decompressed and anchored when the movements and postures of the exercises in this book have become absolutely automatic, when you're no longer "translating" in your head how to hold yourself and move right. You're doing it right without thinking about it—unconsciously if not subconsciously.

Or, by the same token, you know you have restored your body's natural foundation of strength and flexibility when the movements and postures you fell into *before* you began these exercises make you uncomfortable, when flopping into a chair or twisting your neck to look behind you is an anomaly, not normal life. That tells you that, like a foreign language seeping into your subconscious, correct movement has become instinctive—the natural foundation of your body once again.

Getting to that point, however, requires considerably more than regularly practicing the decompression and anchoring exercises in the previous three chapters; it requires making the movements and postures of those exercises daily habit until they become your automatic, unconscious way of holding yourself and moving. Ironically, however, achieving that unconsciousness takes a sustained period of very conscious awareness when you need to be mindful of your movements in just about everything you do—in all the activities of daily living that make up the routine of your day.

This chapter is a guide to how to go about meshing correct movement seamlessly into the daily routine of your life, whether you're at home, at work, on the road, hanging out, or stepping out, morning till night. Certainly, not every suggestion is applicable to every life, but it is hoped that you will adapt what's discussed here to your own situation. The point is that how you hold yourself and how you move when you do what's ordinary—whether it's sitting at a desk or waiting for the bus, driving the kids to school or cleaning the house, walking the dog or checking your email—is what will ultimately restore your body's natural foundation so that you don't have to translate at all to maximize the inherent power and flexibility that come naturally to you.

MOVING MINDFULLY TO MOVE RIGHT

The problem is that while it's certain is that your body's frame needs to be supported through axial-appendicular tension in whatever you ask it to do, the small, simple, typically repetitive activities of daily living you need to concentrate on are precisely the sorts of activities we all tend to perform mechanically—without thought or premeditation or even much energy.

So how do you suddenly imbue these routine tasks with purpose? The easy answer is to tell yourself to focus, to stay aware of what you're doing, to be mindful. But how precisely do you do all that when the brain, so busy organizing, operating, and controlling every function and process of the body, is so apt to wander in a million different directions?

It requires effort. Significantly, it requires the initial effort of forcing that wandering brain to come to rest and focus on your body and how it moves. Unfortunately, the only trick I know of that will do this for you automatically is pain, the subject of the next chapter, for pain is able to remind us all too sharply of how we're holding ourselves and how we're moving. Otherwise, the only way to take control of your consciousness and focus it on meshing particular postures and movements into the mundane activities of daily living is by just doing it. There's no other way except to preplan the intention to focus and carry it forward—and when it gets dropped, as it invariably will, simply to pick it up again without self-recriminations.

What in due course reinforces the intention is that the brain works on the pleasure principle. The more you carry forward the intention to be mindful of how you hold yourself and move through the activities of daily living, the stronger and more flexible your body will become and the better you will feel. The pleasure you take in how you feel in time becomes the incentive to move right, and eventually, moving right becomes your new normal—habitual, automatic, and unconscious.

It will take time. No surprise there; it took years for you to let your body adapt itself into incorrect postures and movements to fit the lifestyle of your time and place. Combating that complacent adaptation with mindful, willful retraining of the way you hold yourself and move won't be an overnight battle.

The goal, therefore, from your first stretch in the morning to your final toothbrushing at night, is mindfully to thread the movements of decompression and anchoring into all the ordinary, automatic activities of your life—to fill your life with them so that they become second nature for your body wherever you are, whatever time it is, whatever activity you are engaged in.

Granted, if you work in an office, it's not always possible to get up from your desk chair and hurl yourself down onto the floor for an anchored bridge posture. A couple of lunge decompressions performed on the sidewalk would probably draw the kind of interest you would rather not attract. And your fellow moviegoers are unlikely to be pleased if you suddenly rise up, crawl over their knees, and launch yourself into woodpecker in the theater aisle. But the truth is that while a half hour spent doing the exercises in this book is a great start on unwriting the effects of compression, it's just the opening chapter. As author of the new message you're sending to your physiology, you have to live the movements till they become the complete manuscript of your body's new foundation.

STARTING YOUR DAY

Good morning—and hold it right there.

We Americans tend to rush things in the morning. We talk about "leaping" out of bed, "racing" to start the day, "wolfing down" a quick breakfast. Try not to. Slow down instead and pay attention to your body, to waking it up and giving it a good start by focusing on how you move, even while still in bed, how you get up from the bed, how you support yourself as you go through the morning's ablutions, through the process of getting dressed, through all the small rituals and habits that are your way of preparing for the day. Do this slowly and carefully, and everything you do for the rest of the day will go much better, I promise.

Start the minute you awaken. Your eyes are open, and you feel an urge to stretch. Good! Make it a supine decompression. Zip your legs together so that your heels, toes, and knees touch one another, and reposition your body long in the spine. Now take about ten decompression breaths.

Focus on keeping your chest big. Again, picture your lungs: They are balloons within your ribcage, and you want to fill them up. Your chest's inhalation circumference is the measure of this, so fill your lungs high and wide and watch the chest get bigger and bigger. Hold that circumference on the exhale, keeping your chest big as you recruit those muscles below the ribcage to maintain support.

Want to get up? Fine. After those ten decompression breaths in the supine decompression posture, sit or stand, face your feet forward, and do ten more breaths either as seated decompression from a chair or from the side of the bed or as standing decompression.

Spend a total of maybe 3 minutes doing these decompression breaths and you will have made a very good start to the day. You will have oxygenated your body, fired up your body's metabolism, activated the muscles all around the torso to get them going on their support function, reminded the spine that it is free to focus on neural

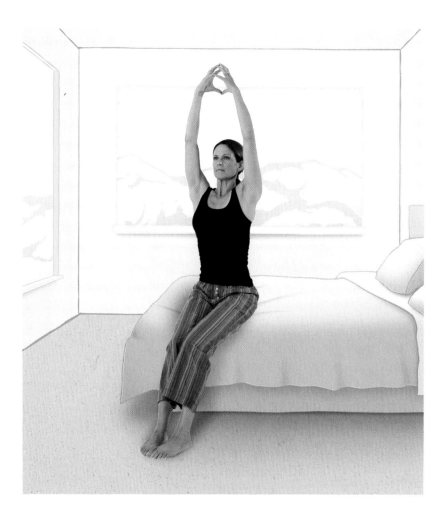

communication instead of having to hold you up, and stimulated your respiratory, cardiovascular, muscular, and digestive systems.

Next step: Head for the bathroom; it's time to wash your face and brush your teeth, not—as may have been your habit—by leaning against the sink in that half sleep you once trudged through knowing that the porcelain would hold you up, but by using the ablutions ritual as an opportunity to strengthen the posterior chain. Seize the

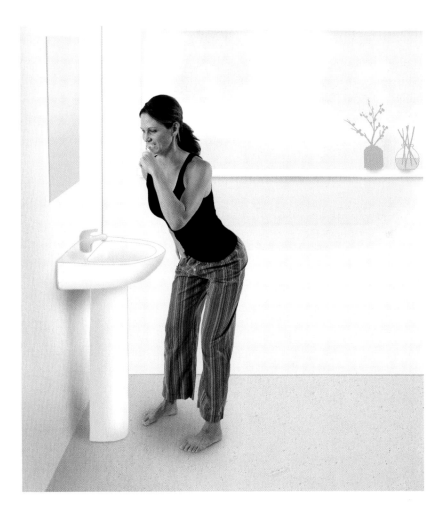

opportunity by spending 30 to 60 seconds of your face-washing time in the founder posture. Return to an upright position to towel off your face by all means, but position yourself in founder for another 30 to 60 seconds while you're brushing your teeth. Stretch the hip joint back as far as you can, lengthening your spine and challenging your posterior chain with every splash of water or mouth rinsing.

It may interest you to know as you do this that, in effect, you're copying or imitating what just about all four-legged animals do when they yawn and stretch simultaneously—it's called pandiculation—a reflex action thought to refresh muscles by stimulating the lymphatic system. You're achieving all that while re-patterning your hip joint through an integrated hinge, activating your posterior chain, and gaining a clean face and teeth.

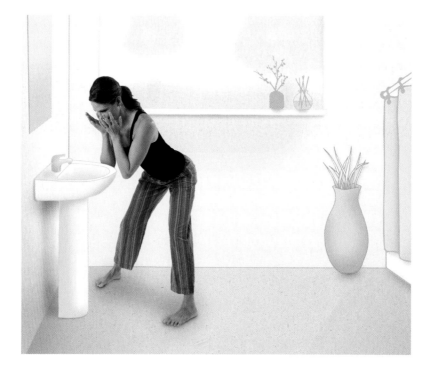

Speaking of "clean," you may be in the habit of running a vacuum cleaner or carpet sweeper here and there around the house before heading out. Each of these is an activity tailor-made for continuing the integrated hinge while adding the counterbalancing movement of your arms reaching forward. The job of vacuuming is particularly suited to starting off in the woodpecker stance, then lunging forward as you push and pull the machine. The woodpecker rotation works great when you need to shift the cleaning head slightly to get into some tight spaces.

No doubt you will need to remind yourself at first—even compel yourself—to position your body in these postures and to execute these movements as you go about doing things that have been utterly mindless up to now. After all, you're at home, it's morning, you're barely thinking as

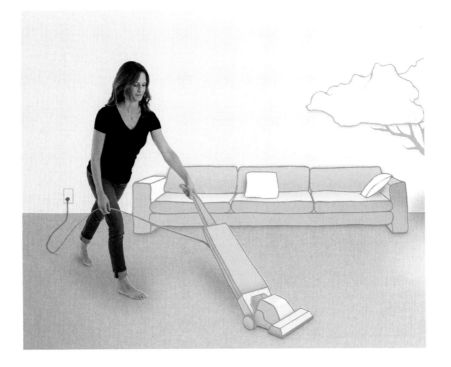

you go through the motions of getting up and getting going. But focusing your mind on small efforts throughout the day can ensure that your body does not regress to default patterns of no resistance. Keep on reminding and compelling yourself till these postures become the new automatic.

COMMUTING

More than 86 percent of Americans commute to and from work by car, van, or truck; 76 percent of us do so as solo drivers.[*]

Just consider: The right foot is pressing the gas pedal so that the foot and leg are always externally rotated. The hip flexors and chest are squashed. The ribcage is pressed down toward the pelvis, while the head is thrust forward in that Queen Nefertiti position called anterior head carriage, with all the ills that can result when the back of the neck becomes shortened and flops onto the neck. It's worth mentioning yet again that such compression can have a seriously unhappy impact on the vagus nerve, and since the vagus nerve is responsible for keeping your heart rate constant and for the process of digestion, you really don't want any kind of impact on it at all, much less a seriously unhappy impact. And that means that as best you can, you want to keep your neck muscles long and your head positioned for space at the back of the skull.

Now let's be clear: When you're behind the wheel of a car, you're

[*] Brian McKenzie and Melanie Rapino, "Commuting in the United States: 2009 American Community Survey Reports," U.S. Census Bureau, ACS-15, September 2011, http://www.census.gov/prod/2011pubs/acs–15.pdf.

there to drive. Safety, obviously, comes first, and alertness is the first rule of safety. Whatever you have to do to stay aware and alert is your first priority; everything else is a distant second. But to whatever extent you can manage it, you will be doing yourself a favor when you press the back of your neck against the headrest put there for whiplash protection and keep your upper back pushed back against the seat. You want your chin to be over your sternum, not ahead of it, if possible. And you should try to keep both feet facing forward and your knees turned toward one another as much as possible. In this posture, you are fighting both external rotation and anterior head carriage. It's a kind of vehicular version of the seated decompression

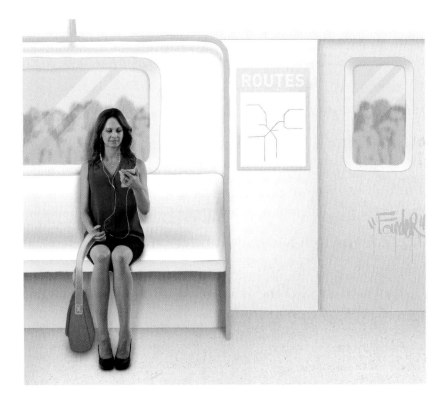

posture—a way of fusing Foundation Training into the realities of our car culture.

Even before you get into the car or train or bus or boat that takes you to work, do three deep decompression breaths in the founder or standing decompression positions. Then, whether you drive to work or are conveyed by a train engineer, bus driver, boat captain, or airplane pilot, think of the commute as a form of seated decompression that you can control.

By the way, if you're in the passenger seat of a car, the seatback and headrest typically make an excellent surface to engage your back as you do frequent decompression breaths. Driving or riding, whenever you can—and certainly if you are stuck in traffic or stopped at a light—do the decompression breath several times for anywhere from 30 to 60 seconds. Similarly, when you can, contract every muscle in your body and hold the contraction for 10 to 15 seconds. These are static holds: Nothing really moves; just contract, then relax. Both actions help your body stave off the worst effects of the enforced compression that driving or being a passenger in some kind of conveyance represents.

And getting into whatever means of transport you use, take three decompression breaths in the founder or standing decompression positions after you exit. It's a great way to undo whatever decompressing the body has just experienced. No one will notice. There's nothing to notice except a person breathing.

Maybe you cycle to and from work. After all, among all commuting modes, bicycling shows the biggest rate of increase nationwide[*]—just

---

[*] Brian McKenzie, "Modes Less Traveled: Bicycling and Walking to Work in the United States: 2008–2012," U.S. Census Bureau, American Community Survey Reports, May 2014, ACS-25, http://www.census.gov/hhes/commuting/files/2014/acs–25.pdf.

ask the residents of Portland, Oregon. But if you commute by bike, you are likely angled forward at about 45 degrees—maybe even less—which makes it natural for you to lean your body weight forward as well. That probably means your ribcage is scrunched inward and your chin jutted outward. You're curled down; you're probably uncomfortable; and the fact is that you are exerting a lot of effort to little effect, in a posture that squeezes your body and in no way positions you to burn as many calories as you should no matter how much huffing and puffing you do. Again, that's the position that seems to come naturally when cycling, but it's a compressing posture you can do something about.

Of course, safety comes first on a bike as it does behind the wheel of a car, but the key here is to make your hips the center and starting point of your movement. Start pedaling from the hips, not with the knees, not in the quads, not anywhere else. To do so, press each foot full-force into the pedals and keep your knees close together and close to the center of the bike—so close that they are almost kissing with each pedal stroke. This positioning, with the balls of your feet and your toes and knees all moving toward the center of the post, primes your gluteal muscles to lift your torso so you widen and lengthen your upper body.

Now you're in the right posture to do what you know how to do: Expand your upper back, pull your neck long, extend your shoulders wide, pull your elbows away from each other. You don't have to change your angle for any of this; just expand and elongate where you are. The idea is for your chest to be up and over the handlebar, so that when you look up, you are doing so with your chest, not your nose.

I can sum it all up best in the immortal words of my friend Peter

Park, a world-class and world-famous personal trainer and a passionate and expert cyclist. He offers a simple and succinct mantra for how to position yourself on the bike: "Break the handlebars," says Peter. What he means is: Bend it like you're a strongman who can tie it into a knot.

I know it's a steering mechanism but pretend it's precisely an iron bar and you're Mr. Muscle Beach (even if you're a Miss, Ms., or Mrs.) in a 1958 cartoon about the feeble wimp who wants to bulk up so he can win the girl. Grip the handlebar with the pinky side of each hand down and the thumb side up and press downward, applying all the force you can to bend that handlebar and turn it into a corkscrew. The action of bending the bar is both static—it's an action, not a movement—and isometric—yes, the bar is pressing back. That means that the force is transferred through your wrists into your forearm and upper arm muscles, and since those muscles are also static and un-moving, the force travels right up the arm into the shoulders, neck, and ribcage. And that's the bottom line, for as you try to bend the handlebar, your shoulders, neck, and ribcage should expand and lift. What you're doing, in other words, is making your body as big as you can get it while riding a bike by pressing down on the handlebar and lifting up in the torso.

That's admittedly a lot to keep in mind as you cycle—especially if you commute to or in a busy city and must concentrate on traffic, stoplights, and other realities—but as you make these adjustments, you will find that you also improve your balance on the bike, find your true center of gravity, burn more calories than before, and boost the efficiency of your pedaling.

AT WORK

We work in office parks and on factory floors, in cubicles or alongside assembly lines, in elegant corner suites or open-space "bullpens," but wherever we work, 86 percent of us, according to a 2013 study,* do it sitting down all day, every day. That has to stop.

I understand that staying glued to your desk can be a point of pride. I understand also that office traditions or office politics may make it expedient to concentrate hard on the task at hand—or to look like you're focused, in any case. But add the hours seated at work to the time you spend seated at meals, the time you spend seated to read or watch television at night, the time you spend seated going through emails or surfing the Internet or playing at your Wii or Xbox or PlayStation, and you will have spent most of your day succumbing to being pressed down into a chair by gravity.

There's a simple solution. At least every 30 minutes—every 20 minutes is preferable—stand up. Don't *just* stand up, either; take a break from work. That is, do something else—something other than work—and what I am going to suggest is a 3-minute decompression routine that will pull your torso up, anchor your pelvis from below, and decompress you. Here it is—five movements:

1. A standing and/or lunge decompression (pp. 50 and 52)
2. A founder and/or integrated hinges (pp. 84 and 90)

---

*Lindsay Olson, "Sitting Disease: The Slow, Silent and Sedentary Killer of the American Workforce," *U.S. News & World Report*, August 22, 2013, http://money.usnews.com/money/blogs/outside-voices-careers/2013/08/22/are-you-suffering-from-sitting-disease.

3.   A woodpecker and/or lunge decompression (pp. 86 and 52)

4.   15 to 20 decompression breaths (p. 44)

5.   Shoulder tracing (p. 62)

By all means, mix it up—in terms of selection and sequence—so long as you do at least 15 deep decompression breaths. Whatever movement or movements you perform, know that each is a physical meditation in which you create stimulation within your body; that is why the three-minute break is so powerful.

And it is why you must be willing to step away from the desk. Especially if you're someone who works at a keyboard staring at a computer monitor in order to execute your job, the break every 20 minutes or half hour is essential. Will your actions strike your fellow workers as odd? Isn't that their problem? Still, if it is awkward for you, there may be a break room or quiet area you can escape to for the three minutes—even the ladies' or men's room. But if it's impossible in some way or for some reason for you to do the routine I've suggested, then at least do something else: Walk to the water cooler, do the decompression breaths, stretch, anything other than sitting. And if there is some impenetrable reason why you cannot take a legitimate work break for three minutes every half hour, have your boss call me because there is something seriously unbalanced either in the organization you work for or in your life, and something must be done about it.

In addition to taking breaks that count—not as a replacement for them—there is also a way to make sitting "pay," and that's by decompressing as well as you can while you're seated. Remember also that you can augment the benefits of these seated decompressions by simultaneously squeezing a water bottle, rolled-up sweater, box of tissues, or the like between your knees as you breathe.

The situation is slightly different if you work in a factory or plant rather than in an office, but what holds true whatever your work environment might be is that spinal stability stems from how you position your ribcage and torso. If your job has you working up against a table where the tendency is to press your hips against the table to rest them, counter that tendency by pulling your hips back and keeping your chest up and over your workstation. If your work requires lifting and/or reaching overhead, counterbalance the lift by squatting, and turn the reach into a lunge or standing decompression. These are easy solutions, and the beauty part is that doing them just looks like you're working—which you are, but you're re-patterning your movements and decompressing your body at the same time.

AROUND THE HOUSE

Being at home typically entails a number of small chores we tend to do mindlessly, but these chores are actually a great target for making the postures and movements of Foundation Training habitual. In most such chores—straightening up a messy room, dusting, doing the laundry, and everybody's least favorite chore on earth, emptying the dishwasher—the key is to focus on integrated hinging. So as you begin to reach down to pull the plates out of the dishwasher, or to look deep in the fridge, or to toss another wet load into the dryer—focus on keeping your feet parallel with your weight on the heels and your toes gripping the floor, as you breathe deeply and hinge at the hip, keeping your spine long and pulling your hips back behind the heels.

Another at-home activity, although it's one you do outdoors, is gardening. Those who are passionate about it can spend endless hours preparing soil, planting, weeding, dead-heading, and more, and I have seen gardeners contort their bodies into absurdly uncomfortable, unflattering, and unhealthy positions. The solution is the posture called kneeling decompression, both

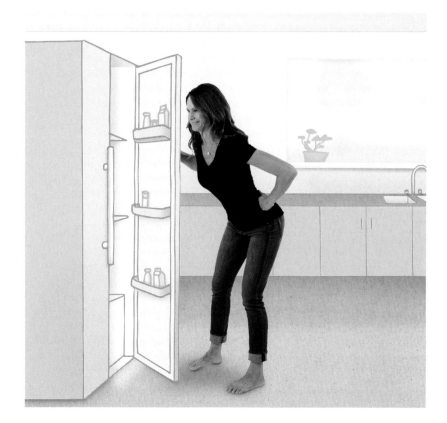

the easiest and the most effective way to execute just about any task in any part of the garden in any season.

Get on your knees but positioned as tall as you can be, with your feet straight back behind you. Make sure all the weight is on the knees, not on the feet; if the weight goes through your feet and your feet grab the ground, that contracts the muscles on the front of your legs, and that, in turn, tightens the abdomen. Instead, keep the weight on the knees, take a deep decompression breath, and hinge your hips back. You're now perfectly positioned for both decompressing and gardening.

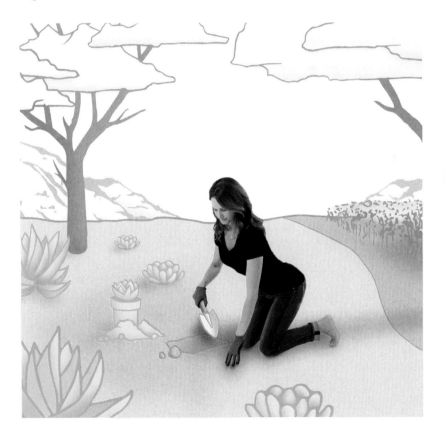

DOWNTIME

You're at the bus stop . . . in line at the deli counter waiting for your order . . . marking time in the lobby till the elevator arrives . . . *in* the elevator, riding up or down: It's time you can use to be as active as possible with as little movement as possible—a great opportunity to activate muscles isometrically, the perfect opportunity to fine-tune your standing decompression posture.

For all intents and purposes—and to all appearances—you're just standing there. But in fact, this is the time to breathe full into your lungs—front, back, sides—raising your sternum, drawing your chin back to keep your neck long and to position your head for space at the back of the skull. Be sure to use your foot muscles as well. Squeeze your feet together and flex and extend your toes inside your shoes.

Downtime is not an annoyance when you use it to improve your health.

EXERCISE AND SPORTS

From professional athlete to weekend warrior, it is axiomatic that the better your body supports itself, the more efficiently it works and the less prone it will be to injury. That's just common sense; such a body is stronger and more flexible and therefore better equipped to sustain physical activity and to withstand physical impact. That is why it is so important to take a decompressed, anchored body into whatever sport or form of exercise you make part of your life.

After all, we all know you can't strengthen the body's foundation by just doing cardio, or just going for muscle mass, or, a little like Hallie back in Chapter 2, just crunching like crazy to sculpt six-pack abs. In truth, you can't do it by just carving out a half hour in which you slip into designated workout garb and head for the gym—although a gym workout is a very good thing to do, as are cardiovascular exercises, weight lifting, and, in moderation, sit-ups. In fact, whether fitness buff or sportsman—or both—whether heading out to the golf course on the weekend or putting yourself through a weekday workout at home or in the gym, there are two things you cannot do without: 1) the right equipment and 2) a warm-up routine. Foundation Training provides both.

The equipment is the body you bring to your favorite sport or exercise. Whether you are going for a layup or going for a walk, swinging a club or a bat or a stick, leaping hurdles or bracing for defense, the body you bring to it should be one that moves correctly and is in sync with its natural capabilities. That general rule applies to any game or exercise.

And as everybody from professional athlete to weekend warrior knows, it's important to warm up before you start your favorite game or exercise. The problem is that too often warming up begins and ends with some sort of hustling move aimed solely at raising the heartbeat—and that simply isn't enough. What your warm-up should do is turn on the right muscles and turn off the wrong ones; that means focusing on those movements that get the biggest muscles in the body equipped and ready to support the big movements your sport or workout will demand of you. So it's not just about getting the heart pumping; it's about stretching and activating the muscles that control your hips, because the hip joint will be at the center of those movements. Whatever your preferred physical activity—heli-skiing or hockey, surfing or soccer, basketball, gardening, track, free-climbing, or raking leaves—if you are going to spend time and effort doing it, you may as well prime your body to gain back as much benefit and gratification as you can from the time and effort you spend.

THE FOUNDATION TRAINING WARM-UP

Each of the exercises in this warm-up routine stands alone as a challenge to your body, summoning it to pull out of its old patterns and into a new one. All of them access the important muscles of the posterior chain. They also prompt you to stretch the muscles along the inner thigh—not so far that they actually weaken, just far enough for them to remain strong as they pull the thighs back toward the center of the body.

Take your time with these exercises; focus on each one to the point of exhaustion. Give your body the chance to become more sensitive to all the muscles you are using *while* you exercise, not just to the muscles that are the object of the exercise.

FOR FITNESS WORKOUTS

Here's a routine especially suited for yoga, Pilates, barre, dance, gyrotonics, or other similar practices that address the whole body. Do each exercise three times for 1 minute each time:

Prone decompression (p. 56)

Anchored extension (p. 78)

Founder, with your legs as far apart as you can comfortably distance them, and focusing on being anchored (p. 84)

For practitioners of CrossFit and for weight lifters, whatever the style of weight lifting and whatever the form or size of the weights, do these four exercises twice each, taking from 30 seconds to 1 minute for each exercise:

Internal leg tracing (p. 70)

Anchored bridge (p. 76)

Shoulder tracing in the founder posture (p. 62)

Shoulder tracing in the woodpecker posture (p. 88)

FOR THE GAMES PEOPLE PLAY

It's hard to come up with exact figures, but among the American populace, men and women both, the competitive games most frequently played are golf, tennis, soccer, hockey, basketball, and baseball, while an estimated 15 million of us pursue the solitary "sport" of running or jogging. All of these sports—in fact, all the sports you love to play—require a warm-up beforehand, whether you're under-taking a training session or practice or actual competition. Such a warm-up should include these five exercises done three times each for 1 minute apiece:

Standing decompression (p. 50)
Lunge decompression (p. 52)
Internal leg tracing (p. 70)
Woodpecker (p. 86)
Founder (p. 84)

For fitness or for fun, whenever you ask your body to work harder than normal, to achieve a level of performance and expend an amount of effort and energy beyond the norm, you need to help it get ready to do so. These warm-ups center the body structurally, ensuring that the muscles central to your hip function are working well so that when you swing the bat, make the leap, lift the weight, slam the return, it is the pelvis that is initiating the motion, giving both your body and your sport the most benefit possible.

ENDING YOUR DAY

Day's end: Work is done, dishes are done, kids are asleep, and you're winding down. That doesn't have to mean that your body is collapsing. Before you turn in for the night, take time for the supine decompression, for in that posture you're still asking your muscles to stabilize even though you're "just" lying there. Hold the posture for 5 minutes while you breathe gently: Inhale through the nose for 5 seconds, exhale through the mouth for 6 seconds. The slightly longer exhalation has long been known in yoga and other Eastern health practices as a calming and destressing influence, and it is a great way to prime the body for a restful sleep—another one of the many valuable lessons I learned from Dr. Tim Brown.

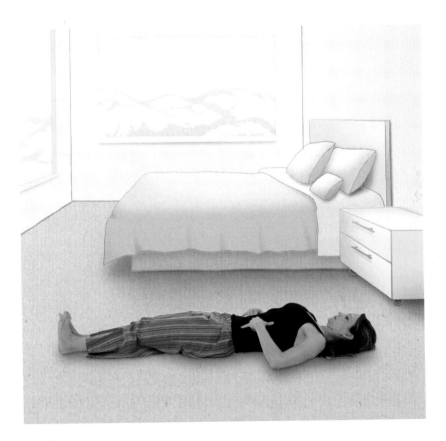

PERPETUAL AWARENESS

Until correct movement is embedded in your unconscious, awareness of your body's posture is both a means and an end in creating new patterns of movement and strengthening your body's foundation. Such awareness is gained through practice, self-reminders, reminding one another if there's a spouse or partner you can turn to in this endeavor. You simply have to be mindful of where you are and what you are doing—and how you are positioned structurally and moving muscularly as you do it.

So there you are watching television in the evening, and you're more or less curled into the couch and scrunched from head to toe. At every commercial break, remind yourself to stand up, decompress, move, activate your muscles before you plop back down.

When you're walking, whether to get somewhere fast or out for a stroll, be aware of how you're doing it. Don't lead with your chin. Actively pull your sternum up and out. Keep your feet pointed straight ahead; that is, after all, where you want them to take you.

You're seated with friends in a restaurant or bar . . . you're at the movies . . . you're in a meeting. Whatever the situation, there is a moment in which you can take control of the way you are holding yourself, raise your sternum, elongate your torso, anchor your feet into the floor, and breathe high, wide, and fully. As you fill your lungs with oxygen, you also fill your life with a new pattern of support that is really a return to your body's natural flexibility and inherent strength.

To make Foundation Training most effective and long lasting, it should be used in your everyday movements. The basic things we do throughout our days can begin to build us up instead of constantly breaking us down. To help you with this, we created the following whimsical story of how Hallie's daily activities incorporate the exercises and keep her free from pain. . . .

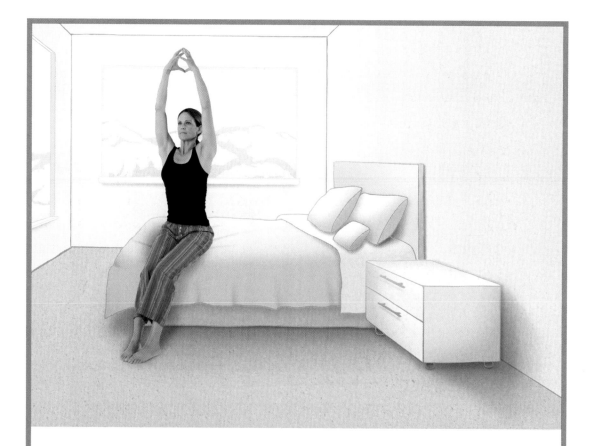

A quick decompression
to start the day.

———

A few focused breaths
and she's well on her way.

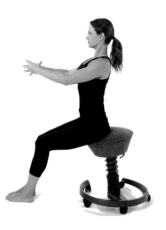

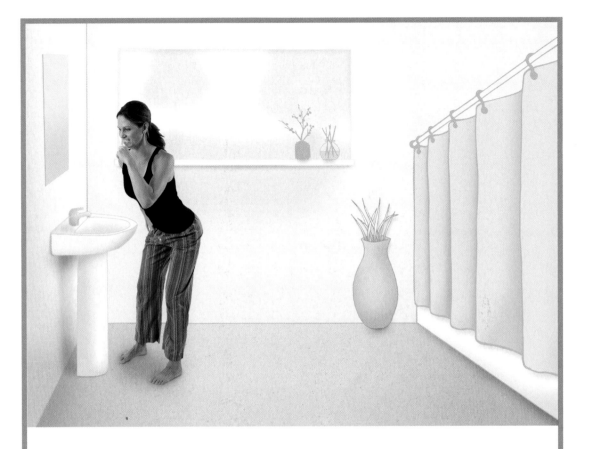

While she brushes her teeth,
she can strike a strong pose.

The founder builds strength
from her head to her toes.

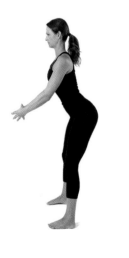

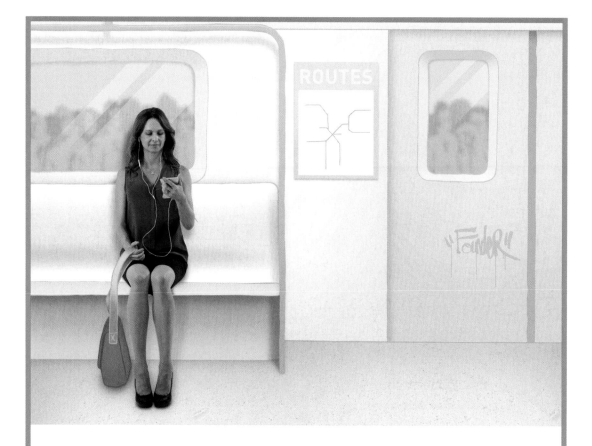

Trains and planes and automobiles
offer opportune times
to press weight through her heels.

———————

Decompression while seated
in her favorite style,
and Hallie stays strong
mile by mile.

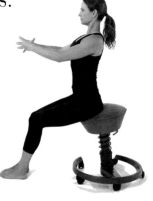

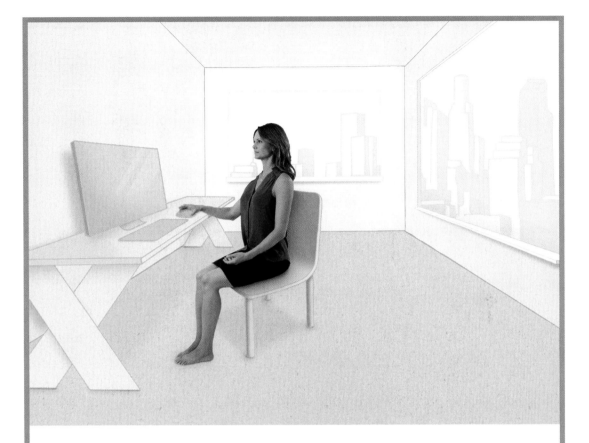

Meetings and emails
set the pace of her day.

———

Some seated decompression
keeps her back pain at bay.

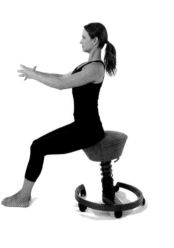

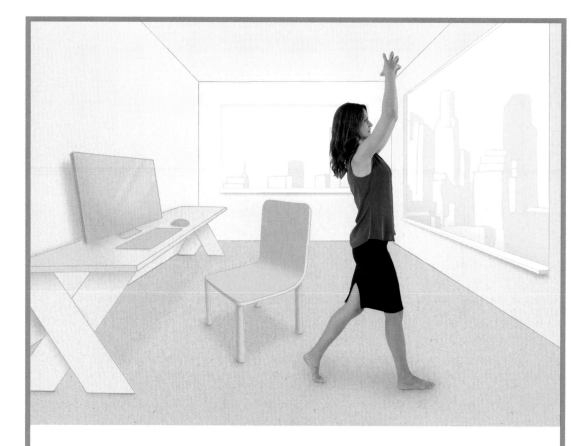

Every 20 minutes
and she's out of her chair.

She stretches hard for a minute,
and fills her ribcage with air.

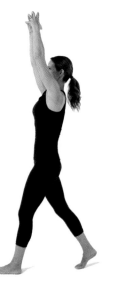

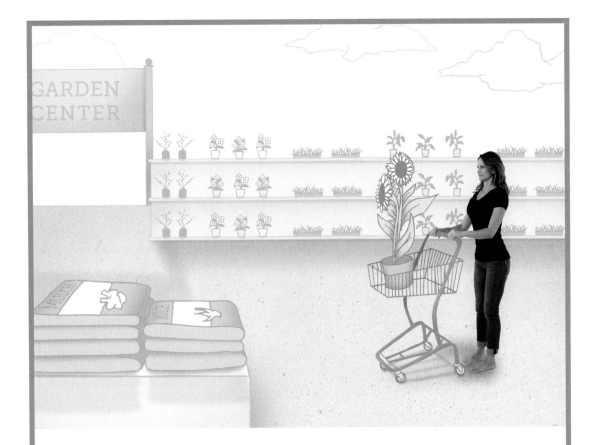

When shopping for shrubberies
or plants big and small.

Hallie keeps in her mind
to stand big and tall.

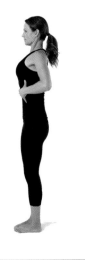

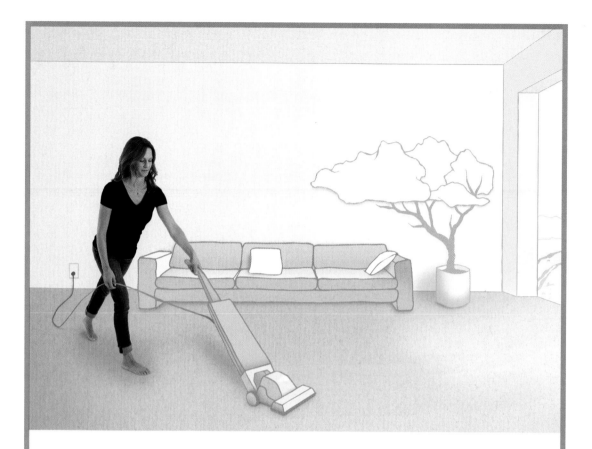

Vacuuming sucks,
but it needs to be done.

———

Hallie uses the chore
to strengthen her buns.

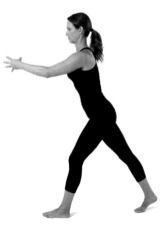

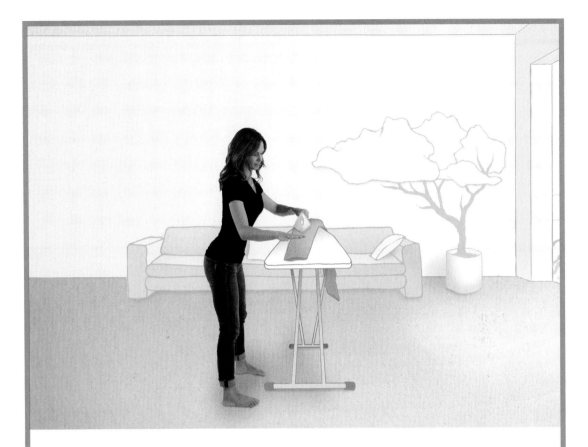

When she irons her clothes
to release all the folds.

———

She knows she'll feel good
from the poses she holds.

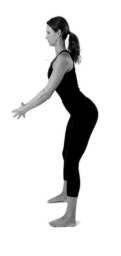

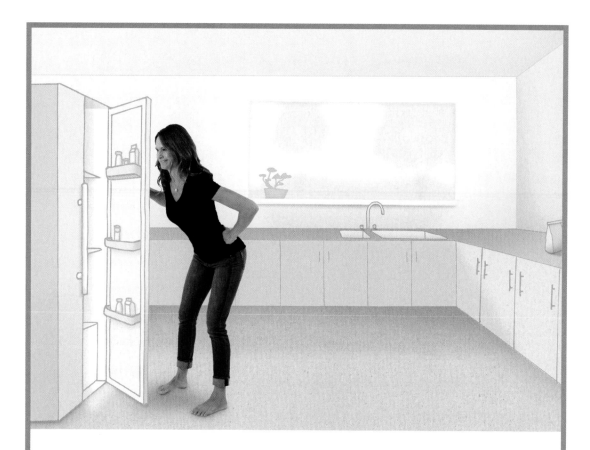

Off to the kitchen
for a snack or a drink.

It's the perfect chance
to strengthen weak links.

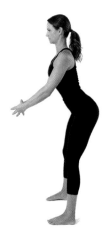

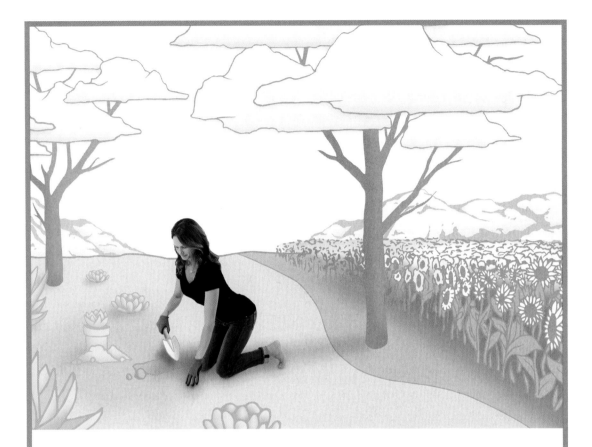

Tending to trees or flowers
or bushes or weeds.

———

A kneeling decompression
suits most of her needs.

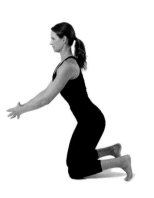

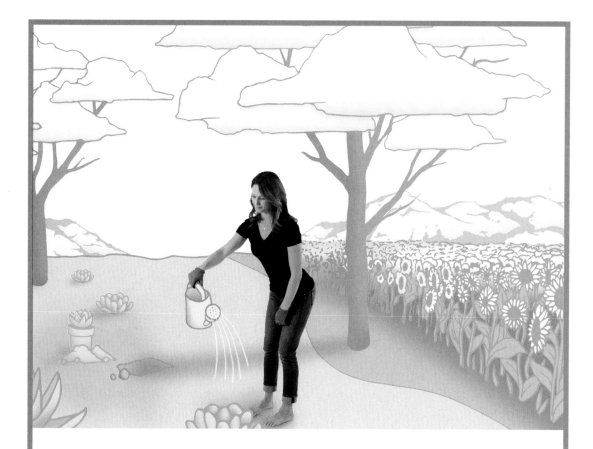

Watering plants at
chest height or below.

She hinges, saves her back,
digs her heels, plants her toes.

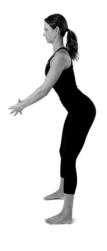

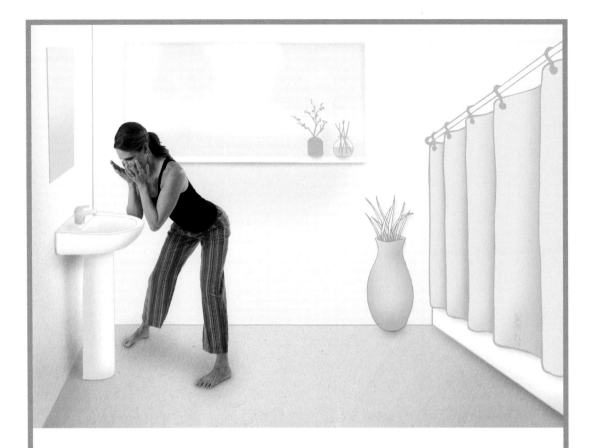

Back to the baño,
to rinse off her face.

As with brushing her teeth,
give her torso some space.

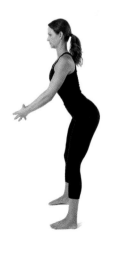

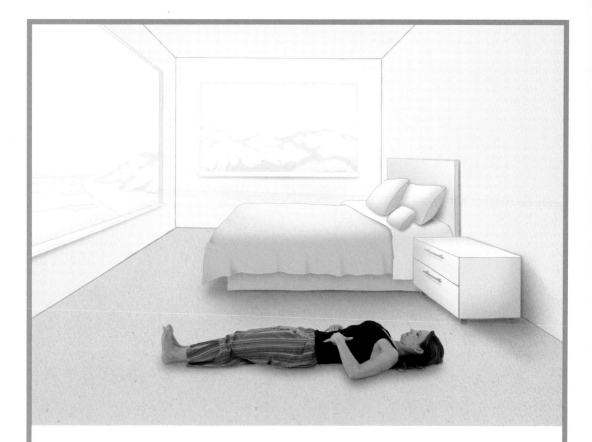

Now done with her day,
to center her head.

Just a brief decompression
and then off to bed.

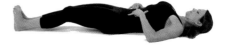

SEVEN

MOVING PAST THE PAIN

A classic bit of knowledge we learn within chiropractic medicine is that mechanoreception blocks nocireception—in plainer English, movement blocks out pain.

Chiropractors aren't the only medical practitioners who know this. It is an understanding common to many branches of health practice, including mainstream medicine, especially among physicians who can acquiesce to patient demands for instant pain relief through drugs while the physicians prescribe rehabilitative movement as therapy.

The goal in this book, however, especially for those of you who come to Foundation Training from a place of pain, is to bring about a more fundamental and profound change in an individual's relationship with pain—not just to put the pain aside but to put it away and move past it. That requires the kinds of foundational change represented in the postures and movements outlined in Chapters 3, 4, and 5. It is change aimed at re-patterning the body back to its natural way of moving, to the baseline from which we have been diverted by our contemporary style of living. It is therefore both radical and comprehensive change.

The change is radical precisely because it must go deep—to the sources and origins of structure and movement in the body's foundation. It is change aimed not at one part of the body or other but at the intersection of the tension between axial and appendicular skeletons—in short, at the wellspring of how the body holds itself. It is fundamental change that targets the origin of movement in the pelvis and not the end points of movement in the limbs.

The change is comprehensive because it enlists the entire body, from head to toe and from inside out of the whole integrated, highly dynamic organism. That's a significant undertaking, with a multiplicity of effects. "Multiplicity of effects" is a shortcut to saying that because the organism is a network in which everything connects to everything else and everything communicates with everything else, wrong movement can make us feel lousy in many ways, not just in muscle aches and pains. And vice versa, to be sure: Right movement can make us feel good in ways that go well beyond strength and flexibility of structure and muscle.

THE NETWORK EFFECT

The biomechanics handled by the outside "wrapper" of the network—the way you move—cannot be dissociated from the neurological messages directing the biomechanics, nor from the bio-chemistry occurring across various organ systems—that is, how the body works and how you therefore feel. And vice versa: The neuro-logical messages and the biochemistry—how the body works and how you feel—show up in how you hold yourself and how you move. No wonder wrong movement causes us pain, and no wonder pain hobbles or distorts our movement. It's a two-way street: Movement writes a message into the body, and the impact of the movement writes a message back. But it isn't just structure and muscles that are affected.

To see the principle in action in a very simplistic way, smile. Turn the corners of your mouth up, flash your teeth, and beam at this book. The odds are good your whole body kind of sat up; your head lifted itself and your torso lengthened and you more or less came to a state of eager attention, ready to go, in a good mood.

Now frown. Turn the corners of your mouth down, bring your lips together in a single, stern line, and scowl. Again, chances are your body slumped, your head dropped, and you began to feel as low, phys-ically as well as mentally, as your sagging face suggested.

This is a not very scientific way of showing you just how quickly the way you feel takes somatic form in the integrated network that is your body. Movement—even movement as small as a smile or frown—inscribes itself into your body. Then the effect of what has been inscribed comes right back down the two-way street and gets written into all sorts of functions and activities going on in the physiology of the body.

My favorite anatomy specialist, Thomas W. Myers, gives the example of how depression changes physiology. First, says Myers, our nervous system translates the low spirits into tightened movement—what he calls "a recurrent pattern of contraction"—in the motor system. Over time, Myers goes on, the fascial system—the connective, stabilizing body sheath in which we are wrapped—begins to reflect this pattern; it too contracts, and therefore the body's central cavity shrinks, squeezing all the organs within. This has the effect of lessening our breathing as well, and that of course changes the biochemistry within us, affecting the flow of blood, nutrients, hormones, and waste. Even if the depression ends or is successfully treated with drugs, it doesn't really go away *so long as the habit of movement remains unchanged,* still stuck in the structure of the fascial system and in the pathways within the body.[*]

And so the reverse works as well. If you re-pattern the body's movements to unwrite the effects of compression, for example, the message of the re-patterning gets communicated to the other systems of the body—a rewrite that extends from the fascial wrapper to all those chemical pathways in the fluids to the zillion neurotransmitters flying across neural routes and junctions to the respiratory and digestive and immune systems and more. Once the messages of *decom*pression have spread around the body, all the impacts of compression begin to dissipate, including the pain the compression caused. Your overall health is better, you feel cheerier, and your pain is behind you.

Does this mean you will be pain-free for life if you practice only right movement? Not a chance. One reason is that there simply is no

---

[*]Thomas W. Myers, *Anatomy Trains: Myofascial Meridians for Manual and Movement Therapists,* Kindle ed. (N.p.: Elsevier Health Sciences, 2013), p. 35.

such thing; nobody gets through life without pain of various intensities and durations, as I probably don't have to tell you. More to the point, there is a difference between the pain that is a signal from your muscles that you have been a little too demanding and the pain that debilitates, limiting your life. It's that latter pain that fades once you have re-patterned your movements, after which the former kind of pain is almost welcome.

I know this from my own experience. I routinely feel pain when I ask too much of a set of muscles; mostly I look on that pain as a summons to keep on doing what I was doing until—sure enough—the pain goes away as the muscles respond to the effort. This is good pain. But I am literally free of the pain I referred to in the introduction to this book—the back pain and hip pain, closely related twin agonies—that dogged my existence when I was in my early twenties with flare-ups lasting from a week to ten days, pain that constricted my life and at times seemed to govern it. That was bad pain. Over time, I was able quite literally to move my way out of that pain, and to this day I continue to keep it at bay and go past it with every move I make.

THE OTHER THING THAT MUST CHANGE: PERSPECTIVE

The tool for effecting this radical and comprehensive change is of course your own body pushing back against gravity and gaining, or regaining, balance and strength through repeated use of the postures and movements in this book. Overseeing the change, however, and making it last is the brain, which is why a cognitive shift is also essential. By this I mean a true understanding of your own body and an accompanying sense of proportion about the care you take with the way you hold yourself structurally and move muscularly.

Partly that changed perspective is a matter of the mindfulness discussed in Chapter 6, the awareness at all times of just that—how you are holding yourself structurally and how you are moving muscularly. Partly it is a shift from the focus on how you feel to a focus on how you move. Above all, it is a function of the fact that since only you can control the instrument of your postures and movements—your body—you are ultimately responsible for its care.

In a very real sense, paying attention to how you move is as essential an aspect of self-care as is paying attention to how and what you eat, whether you're drinking enough water, keeping yourself and your home clean, practicing personal hygiene—the things we all do so automatically we don't even think of them as self-care. But they *are* aspects of self-care. They are necessary functions for living that are under our control, maintenance functions that we initiate and execute deliberately, and among them is the need to be aware of how we move and, with conscious intention, to move right.

As the three people you will meet in this chapter exemplify, the obligation to practice self-care is the key to changing both perspective and body movement patterns, and thus to moving the pain away, getting past it, and moving on.

LIFE IN THE OFFICE

Justina Pham is a dentist who enjoys a successful practice and a successful family life with her husband and two small children. The only smudge in this bright picture is the acute lower back pain that Justina suffered for twenty-three years.

The pain came in episodes that occurred regularly, lasted for days, and were utterly debilitating. Over the years, the bouts of pain had managed to both complicate and limit Justina's confidence in her own strength, to diminish her personal life—for example, interrupting her ability to lift her two young children—and, on an hour-by-hour basis, to adversely impact her professional life in the office where she cared for her patients. Seated most of every day, body angled forward as she stared into patients' mouths and executed delicate techniques to minister to the health of their teeth, Justina wondered whether her pain might at some point put her in danger of doing less than her best for her patients.

This is a health practitioner who could never get a satisfactory answer from her doctors about the cause of the pain. An MRI showed two bulging discs and one herniated disc, but since nothing was impinging on the nerves, Justina knew this could not have been the cause of pain. One doctor told her she had probably fallen on her tailbone as a kid and was suffering for it now. "What kid doesn't fall on her tailbone?" Justina wanted to know, a question that elicited only a shrug from the physician.

She was not the first health practitioner to be frustrated by her profession's inability to deal with what had become a large factor in her life. Nor was she the first to feel that her own pain was diminishing her professional capabilities. "Back pain makes you feel helpless," says Justina. That feeling of helplessness is not uncommon among health-care practitioners and constitutes, in my view, what is and ought to be as serious a concern within the profession as the issue of burnout, to which I am sure it is related. So many practitioners in contemporary health care—from physicians to chiropractors, from physical therapists to dentists—are themselves in pain; not surprisingly, they worry that their effectiveness is reduced by that pain. In many cases, the feeling of helplessness Justina expressed can become a source of guilt, not entirely misplaced: If you are not confident in your own body's well-being, it is not unreasonable to wonder how you can legitimately serve the well-being of your patients.

That is why the changes Justina made in her movement patterns, changes that, in her own words, so "profoundly affected" her entire life, have such wide-ranging implications. For herself, the ability to have put the pain behind her has been significant, and she can see and feel "a huge difference" in the very shape of her body as well as "physically, mentally, spiritually." Freed from fear of those stretches of intense pain that constantly loomed as a possibility, she has moved from helplessness to making movement an obligation of her own self-care, a changed perspective with broad implications for her personal life and professional life as well as for her own sense of well-being.

It is more than just kicking off the day each morning with

decompression breathing and a sequence of Foundation Training postures and movements. Freedom from fear of the "next" episode of acute pain has bred and sustains a new level of confidence in her strengthened body. It means Justina can lift up her children with ease, hinging at the hip to do so—without pain or fear of pain. It also means that the way she sits as well as how she is standing or walking or moving at all are constantly, in her words, "in the back of my mind." These days Justina's focus in her individual movement practice is to work with her instructor to modify some movements she finds problematic—to "do movements that I feel are safe for me" and that, in her view, enable her to strengthen herself "without worry."

But it is perhaps the very practical changes Justina has made in her professional life that are the most profound and influential. In that realm, she has implemented alterations in everything from the office furniture to encouraging her staff toward the kind of self-care she now practices. Where Dr. Pham used to perch on the edge of a chair to examine patients, she now straddles a saddle stool that "keeps me long in the torso." She scheduled in-office sessions for the entire staff with her own certified instructor in Foundation Training movements, sowing the seeds of a similar awareness in her colleagues and employees. She is bringing a new consciousness of movement as part of self-care to practitioners dedicated to caring for others; even dental patients win when practitioners get ahead of their own pain in these ways.

Health-care practitioners have long been advised to "heal thyself."

Here is a health-care practitioner who has threaded that advice into both her personal and professional life in ways that benefit herself, her family, her coworkers, and her patients.

EQUATING PHYSICAL ABILITY WITH SELF-WORTH

For Brian Fishbook, sense of self meant physical prowess, so when the prowess was dented and ultimately shattered, there wasn't much to fall back on. "My outrageous strengths," Brian astutely says, "were keeping me from dealing with my outrageous weaknesses." For Brian, born and raised in beautiful British Columbia, Canada, where he skied, hiked, climbed, mountain-biked, and of course played hockey almost as soon as he could walk, those outrageous strengths were natural physical capabilities that made any activity, any sport, any game, any effort a breeze. And that was lucky, because physical activity was what Brian loved. He was simply a natural and passionate athlete and—no way around it—an adrenaline junkie.

It was also central to his profession—ski patrol in the winter and mountain fire corps in the summer, activities dependent on physical strength sufficient to breed a kind of physical and mental fearlessness in the face of risk. Brian relished it all, and he flourished in the culture of toughness-at-all-costs that was the context of his work and a key motivating factor of his life. Brian's physical ability defined him.

So when he blew out his knee at age twenty-three and tore his ACL, his anterior cruciate ligament, in the classic injury that has derailed so many athletic careers, Brian barely slowed down. His solution was "to go harder," to push through. And fortunately, his wonderfully honed body responded easily, recruiting other muscles to compensate for the mechanics the knee once handled, as Brian continued to ski seven days a week, sometimes for twenty-five days at a stretch, and then to rappel out of helicopters to fight fires in the summer. Cool, he thought. I'm good. I will just keep going. The culture, his sense of himself, Brian's whole perspective on life just said: Press on.

So he did. Through groin pain that just kept getting worse, through a chain of discomforts and minor injuries, through cortisone shots and acupuncture, massage and therapy, and through an increasingly downward spiral in his head and his emotions. Why do I find this so difficult? he wondered. Convinced he was only half as tough as everyone else on his crew, a crew he now managed, Brian struggled even harder—and grew even more depressed. He was in his mid-thirties, and the wheels were coming off. When Brian hit his forties, they came off for good.

Two season-ending injuries in a row finally convinced Brian that he needed to make fundamental changes if he was going to bring sanity and well-being back to the way he lived. He was losing the work that was the center of his life, the physical ability that he thought defined him, and his entire sense of himself. A colleague had put him onto Foundation Training, and Brian even got in touch with me via email; I knew where he was coming from, understood the culture of toughness, and most of all, I knew exactly how he felt.

It was the same struggle I had had, the same inability to cross over into the sensation that moving better produces because it just didn't seem tough enough or corrective enough or radical enough to bring back the strength that had slipped away. At the time, we had no certified Foundation Training instructors in Canada, so Brian began working on the practice via Skype. He was in a cast from his second season-ending injury when he began to change his patterns of movement—on the floor, which was all that could be managed due to the cast—but through all that, the work began to make a difference, and Brian hasn't stopped since.

It is safe to say that today, he sees physical prowess in a whole new light. "Push harder" has been replaced by the need to, in Brian's words, "fire up the initial pathways" that can move him into deeper motions. "Keep going" has turned into finding the stance where he is maintaining neutral tension between axial and appendicular skeletons, getting anchored, and breathing in a way that fills his ribcage front and back. "Press on" has become decompression breathing with room at the back of the skull for all those messages to and from his central nervous system. That new perspective on how to define physical ability also reshapes how Brian defines himself and has prompted him to question what else he might not be thinking about in terms of caring for himself. Once he had put the pain behind him, there was a space left where the adrenaline addiction had been; today Brian fills it with his own capability for self-care.

A POST-OP THERAPIST SEEKING TO AVOID SURGERY

"Something was changing." That is what Joseph Paul realized not long before he was to undergo major surgery on his spine. Like Dr. Justina Pham, Joseph is a health-care practitioner. Specifically, he is a physical therapist specializing in pre- and post-operative spine disorders. He became a physical therapist when at the age of twenty-two a bilateral fracture of his lower vertebra—the pars interarticularis— began the process of degeneration known as spondylolisthesis, the forward displacement of a vertebra under the unprotected pressure of gravity, and made it effectively impossible for him to do the manual work he had hoped to do. Joseph went back to school and eventually trained as a physical therapist, qualifying at the age of thirty-five.

A quarter of a century later, when Joseph was in his early sixties, and following an emergency operation to relieve a ruptured disc in his spine (at the L4-L5 level), the spondylolisthesis was sending waves of pain down Joseph's legs and making his life miserable. It was also turning his life's work into an exercise in acute irony—that is, his own situation was as bad as, if not worse than, the often very complicated spinal issues it was his job to treat. Joseph's doctor had recommended double-vertebrae fusion surgery, a procedure difficult to schedule because it is so complex to perform. The surgeon must, in effect, almost literally tear apart the center of the body in order to perform the fusion, moving aside muscles, fascia, and organs.

Joseph knew all about 360-degree two-level fusion procedures, as physical therapists call this fusion surgery. "That's what I treat," he says. "These are the people I work with. I try to get them up and moving again. So I knew what I was in for." As painful as his life had become, he was in no hurry to go through what he calls "the worst horror story ever." Still, Joseph's case went onto the waiting list for the next available surgery slot, not expected for several months.

Meanwhile, he had begun practicing the postures and movements of Foundation Training with a local certified instructor, and despite decades of following the research and trying "everything under the sun," he began to feel what he was certain was a lessening of the symptoms—in particular at first, diminution of the very serious pain in his legs. The longer he kept at the practice, the better he felt. While everything he had tried through the years had helped "a little," in his words, the forward progress never really lasted. This improvement felt different, as indeed it was. Where earlier conventional improvements had masked his pain temporarily, the re-patterning of his movements through Foundation Training was actually reeducating his muscles and making his hip joint the central absorber of gravity's pressure. With two months to go before the surgery, Joseph canceled the operation; the something that was changing was making enough of a difference that he was getting ahead of the pain and leaving it behind him. He believed that what he had learned through changing his body's foundation was the "icing on the cake of everything I know about the spine."

Joseph has since become a certified instructor in Foundation Training and applies it routinely to his patients. "For chronic spine disorders, multisurgery spine disorders, very complicated spine issues," he says, the use of these postures and movements has realized "nothing but positive results." Even when modifying things "to get somebody started," the results are all positive. "We might get somebody sore," says Joseph, "but we're not having any increases in compression syndromes, and as long as we're not doing *that*, we're on the right track."

Here is a veteran physical therapist who has healed himself and turned his self-care right back into his work of healing others, helping them put their pain behind them and move on as he did.

LIFE-CHANGING

In all three of these cases, it's important to note what changed and what didn't. Justina still has bulging discs, Brian's bone structure remains permanently injured, Joseph's body did not rewind to the age of twenty-one, before he, like so many young athletes, suffered the pars fracture. A change of perspective—a change of focus from how they were feeling to how they were moving—initiated the re-patterning of movements that made the difference. They literally moved the pain out of their lives, and they will need to continue the movements that keep it out. For all of them, there can be no recess from the reeducation of their structural and muscular foundation.

Moving past pain is life-changing, but achieving it requires changes in your life—permanent changes in the way you hold yourself structurally, move muscularly, and think about caring for your body and your self.

EIGHT

LITTLE BODIES BECOME
BIG BODIES

Aren't little bodies born with instinctive potential for the correct postures and movements this book wants to train us back to? Indeed they are, but a child's development, which begins way earlier than most of us ever thought, doesn't happen in a vacuum. From the get-go, children mimic their parents. What the adults around them do becomes the stimulus for their own development. So while the inherent instincts for right movement will unfold in little bodies, they can be moderated, modified, twisted, and turned as the little bodies copy the movement patterns exemplified in the big bodies around them.

That is certainly a call to arms for parents—a summons to represent the right patterns of movement to be mimicked, and an urgent suggestion to do even more. In fact, we now know that the first year of life constitutes a beautifully opportune time to help your child develop those muscles that can keep him or her strong for life. We also know that not doing so can lead to problems in both physical and cognitive development pretty early on. Those discoveries are at the heart of the work of licensed physical therapist Jeanene Salas, a specialist in infant movement, who is accustomed to seeing breakdowns in movement in kids as young as two or three. Such breakdowns manifest themselves as imbalances on one side of the small body or the other, asymmetries that are at the core of motor skills problems that can hold back a child's physical and mental development in profound and lasting ways. Clearly, where such imbalances and incorrect movements are concerned, the more time that passes, the tougher it is to undo the pattern and replace it with correct movement.

The key, as Salas and other specialists in infant movement confirm, is to begin imparting or imposing correct movement on a child in infancy, for that is when the imbalances that may lead to later motor skills problems begin. But how can you impart to an infant the principles of right movement that can help him or her confront a lifestyle likely to offer few demands to resist gravity? How can you help a baby build a physical foundation that can fight compression, stay anchored in the tension between axial and appendicular, and initiate movement in the pelvis across a lifetime to come? If it sounds like this means that new parents should become personal trainers to their infants, that's about the size of it.

HELPING FORM THE FOUNDATION

Mostly, the personal training will consist of challenging and providing encouragement for the baby's natural curiosity about the physical world in which he or she has landed. You almost can't start this too early.

Of course, at every monthly checkup, your family pediatrician will be tracking the baby's progress on the expected developmental milestones—rolling over, sitting up, head control, starting to walk, and so forth. What is equally essential is that the baby achieve key motor skills milestones by the time he or she becomes vertical, after which it becomes much more difficult to tease out any asymmetries or imbalances. Keep in mind that it is during this crucially important first year of life that the spine assumes its natural curve, and parents-as-personal-trainers can help with that by applying a mix of stretching, massage, positioning of their infants, and, above all, engaging with the infants in challenging ways so that the babies' bodies recruit the muscles they need and develop those muscles as they should.

For example, you're probably accustomed to placing your baby on her belly during the day so she can look around on her own. She'll peer up, down, and to either side as she explores the environment around her, taking in stimulating impressions that fire up her sensory system. But as she lifts her head, she's also igniting her neck muscles, and that in turn pulls on the bones of the neck, which in turn helps shape the curve of the spine. That's only the beginning. Face, head, neck—development literally goes from head to tail—and in due course, she'll be able to raise her torso as she props herself up on her arms with her elbows bent. This develops her arm muscles and strengthens the back muscles that hold the spine in its natural curve. It all means that by the time she is vertical, she is in balance, and the symmetry will persist as her muscles and bones lengthen as she matures.

That is why any asymmetry in that whole process is so important to note. Perhaps the baby peers only to the right, or presses her ear to one shoulder, or, once she does start to roll over, favors one side over the other. Such asymmetries, tiny as they seem, can follow her throughout the elongation of her muscles and bones, and she will head into verticality off-balance and at risk for motor skills issues that can become embedded in her physical development and can affect her sensory and mental development.

It's why it's so important for parents to be aware of how crucial this early play on the belly is. It is activity that directly develops the muscles of the baby's core, the center of gravity, and the place from which all her movements will originate once she is vertical. Parents must take the time to challenge the baby during this belly play, engaging her as she lifts her head and neck—look this way, then that way, look up, look down—so that she is recruiting and strengthening the muscles that are crying out for development. Continue the engagement as she begins to prop herself up on her palms, probably around month six, seven, or eight, recruiting muscles and developing strength farther down the spine and along the sides of her body. And keep it going as she advances to getting up on her hands and knees as preparation for crawling. All are key stages of development toward curving that spine and getting ready to get vertical, and she should be challenged every step of the way.

Then, of course, you can gently stretch and massage those challenged muscles after their workout, with the kind of loving touching that is also key to a child's development.

By the way, few things are more of a detriment to this development than parents overusing the car seat, the ubiquitous essential that seems to define contemporary parenthood, as a general carrying vehicle. The car seat was devised for a single purpose and should be reserved for that purpose only: travel. It keeps the baby propped up and safe *in the car,* but it also compresses the baby's body and lets his or her head wobble. Check it out next time you're in a supermarket and come upon a baby strapped into a car seat that is in turn stuffed into a market cart, and you'll see what I mean. Secured tightly and slumped down as the baby is, probably at an angle, its body seems to be increasingly scrunched as the cart is pushed along, and the head teeters and sways all over the place. It is a posture that is already compressed and asymmetrical—not the best start to life.

So are parents better off carrying their baby? Yes, and it even offers the opportunity for some resistance training as you lift and hold the bundle that is your child. Once the baby is walking, however, he or she should not be carried too much. Inconvenient as it may be to help a just-walking baby walk when you have chores to do, it's a stimulating challenge to the baby. Every step, every view—whether he is gazing up, or looking at eye level, or examining the floor or path—ignites those sensory stimuli, and getting those stimuli charged while at the same time the baby is resisting gravity makes the walk, slow though it may be for the parent, a plus for the baby's physiological foundation and mental acuity.

From the very dawn of life, therefore, parents have the chance to support and strengthen the patterns of correct movement in tiny bodies just beginning to push back against gravity. It's about the best head start you can give them.

But of course, once kids are walking on their own, they are, in more ways than one, very much on their way out of your hands. They are now striding forward to their own physical development; it is they who control their bodies, and about the best a parent can hope for is to influence that development.

How can you exercise that influence? Your toddler never stops moving. Your preschooler is a bundle of kinetic energy. Kids in the early grades in school are forced to be sedentary for a good part of the day—unfortunately, at a time when their bodies are fine-tuning motor skills, coordination, endurance, and balance. After that, it's all about puberty and adolescence, when pretty much anything you say or do will qualify as irrelevant or as grounds for an argument or a summons to rebellion. So what can parents really do to ensure that their children have the right foundation of balance and correct movement that can spare them the compression their lifestyle will impose? How can you anchor them in the habits that will keep their bodies strong at the core, balanced front to back, supported by the muscles along the posterior chain, with plenty of space for the joints to move as they should?

FOUNDATION TRAINING AT HOME: STRAIGHTFORWARDLY OR BY STEALTH

In some families, it may work to teach the postures and movements of Foundation Training as a discipline the whole family adopts and follows. Movement sessions might be scheduled, with attendance required. After all, you may require attendance at regularly scheduled Friday night dinners at Grandma's, or perhaps the whole family goes to church on Sunday mornings and you require your kids' attendance there, maybe with a dress code requirement thrown in as well. Or perhaps you insist that your kids take music lessons and practice regularly, or you placed them in a day care center where they would be sure to learn Mandarin. There are all sorts of ways you as parents direct all kinds of behavior that you have determined will be an element of your household or a principle of your family life, and Foundation Training can easily fall into that category. As with any practice begun in early childhood, Foundation Training can thereby become ingrained in your kids' lives—at least for as long as they are part of your household and under your watchful eye.

In many households, however, this kind of disciplined approach would be impractical, impossible, or simply not the family's style—too much like imposing a chore, some would say, like the vegetables you have to eat before you can have dessert or the room you have to clean up before you're allowed to go out to play. Do that, these parents feel, and the Foundation Training movements invariably take on the patina of undesirability; they get all tied up with something disagreeable—a task the kids are required to do, like homework. So far from getting ingrained in the kids' lives, proper movement could turn into something tedious they will want to avoid.

One thing parents in such households can count on, however, is that kids are natural mimics. All of the experts consulted for this chapter—experts both as parents and as practitioners of Foundation Training—agree that because their kids more or less automatically follow their lead, they are particularly conscious of setting an example of right movement. They find if they put on a DVD showing a sequence of Foundation Training movements, their children will invariably ape what they are doing. Ditto without the DVD. A parent stopping to do a founder in the middle of the day typically warrants a me-too imitation by the child. Erin Low says her two kids invariably make fun of her when she positions herself—butt extended—to deal with the washing machine, but the kids mirror her action just the same.

"If I'm doing a session by myself," says Dr. Brennan Bates, a sports chiropractor and a certified Foundation Training instructor, "the kids copy me. It's fun for them." He adds that his children—three boys and a girl, all two to three years apart in age—"can do the exercises easily. It's easiest of all for the youngest, who has of course spent less time sitting at a desk. So far, anyway."

All the parents know there is little they can do about the long-term sitting their kids do once they are in school—except perhaps lobby their local school board to transition to standing classrooms, or at least ask the school principal and teachers to consider hourly breaks during which the kids stand and stretch. But they *can* do something about it at home—and they do. Erin Low's son and daughter know they may not sit on the couch with a device—phone, tablet, laptop, game console—and "I try to remind them that when they do sit on the couch, to do so responsibly, holding themselves as decompressed as possible." They've been outfitted with standing desks as well, so they are upright when they're doing homework, with Mom occasionally cueing them about their posture.

It really comes down to that—what another certified instructor, Kim Katerba, mother of four, refers to as "cueing and coaching," and it is the perfect supplement to both scheduled Foundation Training, if that's what your family has opted for, or Foundation Training by stealth. For the truth is that the one thing parents can bequeath to their children—and it is perhaps the most effective tool you can give them—is awareness. "They are aware," says Erin Low, "that gravity is pushing us down. All of us. And they are aware that we must push back. That is a constant in our house."

Often, the cueing and coaching that keep the awareness alive are as simple as telling children to get up, get outside, get active. Go climb a tree, toss a ball, jump rope, play hopscotch, run from here to there. Their bodies are not compartmentalized parts; they're whole bodies, struggling to lengthen and grow and develop, and yearning to move vigorously and energetically. Get them started, and they won't want to stop.

The cueing and coaching also include pointing out their bad posture or wrong movement. It may sound like discipline, but kids take it in. It can be eye-opening for them, particularly as they notice the need for correct movement or improved support in others. Parents may find it rewarding indeed to hear their children commenting on the way others hold themselves or move, or to hear them taking strangers to task for their compressed bodies or off-balance movements. It may be less rewarding when your kids disparage *your* posture or movements, but it's a sign that they've taken to heart precisely what you wanted them to; just as you hoped, awareness of wrong movement—and therefore of right movement—is becoming second nature to them.

DISTRACTIONS AND SPORTS

Certainly, there is a lot going on in your children's lives outside your home—and outside your control—that militate against your efforts to make Foundation Training a family value. School, friends, social pressures, and just plain old kid lethargy can undermine even the strongest sense of awareness in them. Kim Katerba has observed, in fairly wide-ranging experience, that compression seems to really "hit" kids around age eight or nine. It is a time when kids are sitting longer in school and are encountering more demanding intellectual work in the classroom. School in general takes on a more vivid and weighty role in children's lives at this time, and all the awareness you have instilled in them about movement just may not offer enough firepower for them in the face of more time spent sitting rather than moving.

At the same time, it's when kids are around that age—nine, ten, a bit older perhaps—that many schools ask them to identify their sport. If they choose one, that means they are going to practice after school, and what they are practicing is repetitive movement—for the most part without the benefit of a solid foundation of strength at the core, the ability to hinge at the hip, or space at the back of the skull. When competitions are held, the kids often spend hours squeezed into a car or bouncing around in a bus or van. So while school sports may keep kids active and teach them cooperation and sportsmanship, they may not be doing all that much for the kids' physiological foundation.

Sports doctor Brennan Bates agrees. That is why he coaches middle school and high school athletes in doing the founder, hinging at the hip, and initiating movement from their core. He cues student athletes on how and where to position their feet and how to make their movement originate from the center of gravity in their pelvis— whether they are cutting back and forth in soccer, going for a layup in basketball, or staying ready for return of serve in tennis. When one of the four Bates children practices piano, Brennan is there to remind him to keep his butt back and his chest up high. When his daughter practices her ballet lessons, he coaches her in lifting her ribcage, de-compressing her spine, and holding her posture.

Erin Low does much the same. When her son or daughter is at the computer, she reminds them to sit up tall. When one or both of the kids get antsy or irritated, she leads them in a bit of decompres-sion breathing to calm and decompress them on several levels. It is a form of cueing and coaching in the little things, the kinds of things that stick with you—the voice of your mother remembered years later telling you to "sit up straight" or "no ball playing in the house!" Remember?

But big things count too. When her son Carter had trouble learning how to hinge at the hip, Erin found the perfect solution. The founder is now Carter's at-bat position when it's his turn at home plate for his Little League team. "Do a good founder position, Carter," Erin will urge. Carter shoves back his butt, hinges at the hip, stretches his torso, takes a few practice swings, and dares the pitcher with his stare. He is perfectly positioned to knock one out of the park. To steal from a famous poem, "No stranger in the crowd could doubt" that's Carter at the plate!

Cueing and coaching are what parents always do. You do it when you tell your children they cannot have the candy bar today, when you remind them to brush their teeth before bedtime, when you tutor them to say "please" and "thank you" or to give their bus seat to an elderly or disabled person. You do all this cueing and coaching out of love to make their lives better. It comes naturally to you; it's what being a parent is all about. Just as natural and loving is to cue and coach them to be strong, stand tall, not to get boxed in or pushed down but rather to be aware of their bodies as they learn to make all the right moves for their health and their life.

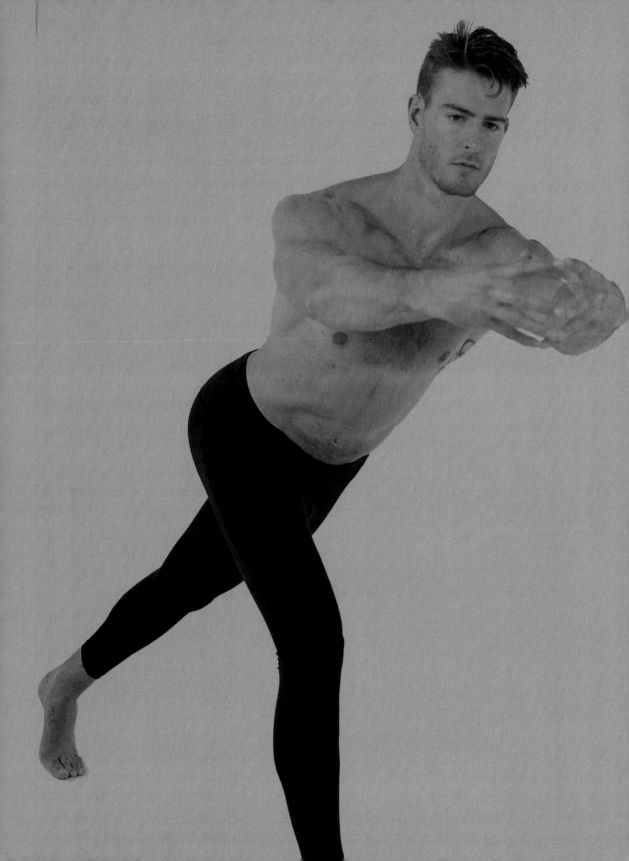

NINE

RETURNING TO THE

FOUNDATION

Remember what compression does to your body's structural integrity? It subverts the push-pull tension between the axial skeleton and the appendicular skeleton and therefore compromises the whole engineering design of skeletal you—the framework of bones connected in such a way as to enable an astonishing variety of movements, the muscles that convert energy into power for both motion and stability, the connective tissue tying it all together, and the fascial wrapper it all comes in.

Obviously, that subversive act also sabotages the purpose that skeletal you is meant to carry out: Maintained by the tension between axial and appendicular, it is the enclosure—the cage—that supports and inspires (literally "breathes life into") the systems of your physiology. Impair it through compression and you do just the opposite: You diminish physiological you and thus handicap your health and well-being.

In fact, right now, to one degree or another, complacent adaptation to the compression of your body under gravity's pressure is adversely affecting processes in some or all of these physiological systems:

- Your respiratory system, because a compressed ribcage limits the lungs' ability to expand and therefore diminishes your breathing, and diminished breathing can unleash a cascade of harmful consequences;

- Your digestive system, because squashed organs don't function nearly as well as they should, and that burdens the body's ability to gain nourishment from food;

- Your circulatory system, because squeezed blood vessels are not as efficient or as effective as they ought to be in transporting nutrients, oxygen, carbon dioxide, hormones, and blood cells to where they need to be transported in order for your body to fight disease and maintain internal stability;

- Your nervous system, because a compressed spinal cord and constricted neural pathways slow the progress of all those neurotransmitters trying to communicate from the periphery to the central nervous system—and back again—and can undermine the brain's ability to coordinate and influence all the activities of your body.

You can change all this and begin to reverse the ill effects that may have come from this compression by relearning how to hold yourself structurally and how to move muscularly. The aim is simply to return your body's foundation to its natural strength and flexibility. It has been the argument of this book that such a return is eminently doable and is an objective for which each of us is perfectly equipped, the main mechanism of the return being the body itself.

To get the process going, start small, stay basic, and do it every day.

SMALL DAILY DOSES

The routine outlined in this chapter is aimed at just that—getting you going on Foundation Training so you can restore your own inherent strength and flexibility, still latent at the core of your compressed body. The routine takes about 10 or 15 minutes; at either length of time, that's a small dose. The watchword, however, is frequency. Success in this case is not dependent on how long you practice a Foundation Training sequence, nor on how intensively you execute each "exercise." It stems from how often you repeat the postures and movements. Frequency of repetition, a steady reminder of how to move correctly, is what teaches the body—just as frequency of repetition is what taught your third-grade mind the multiplication tables or your high school mind the lines of your part in that play you were so good in. That is why the name of the game is to commit to this small dose of movement for this short period of time every day. It is your best shot at sustaining pain relief and establishing the level of fitness you want for your life. Once a day will do it. Twice a day is even better.

Over the course of six days—Monday through Saturday (or however you like to schedule your week)—the routine will take you through pretty much all fifteen of the postures and movements described in Part 2 of this book. The instructional photos are repeated here for your easy reference. On the seventh day, a day typically for recreational and family activities, you'll focus on integrating what you've repeated during the week into precisely those kinds of activities—the activities of daily living. Here's how it works:

Monday, Wednesday, Friday 3 repetitions of each	Tuesday, Thursday, Saturday 3 repetitions of each
1. Standing Decompression	1. Supine Decompression
2. Lunge Decompression	2. Prone Decompression
3. Woodpecker	3. Founder
4. Internal Leg Tracing	4. Woodpecker
5. Anchored Bridge	5. Woodpecker Rotation
6. Anchored Back Extension	6. Integrated Hinges
7. Kneeling Decompression	

1. Standing Decompression

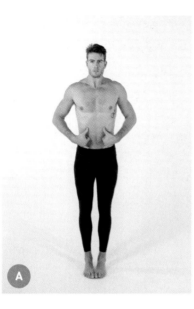

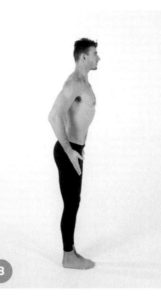

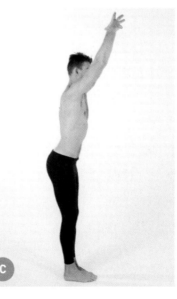

A. Stand tall with the ball of the big toes touching each other and the heels 1 inch apart to line up your pelvis.

B. Open the arms with the elbows slightly bent. Use the upper back and mid-back muscles to expand your chest. Thumbs point away from each other.

C. Lift the arms without straining your neck. Push the crown of your head back and up as the arms lift. Expand the torso and press the ball of the big toe into the ground.

MONDAY, WEDNESDAY, FRIDAY · THREE REPETITIONS OF EACH

2. Lunge Decompression

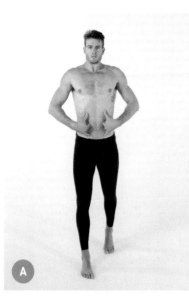

A

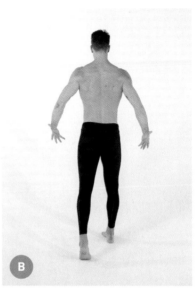

B

Stand tall with the ball of the big toes touching each other and the heels 1 inch apart to line up your pelvis.

A. Stand tall with one leg in front of the other in a strong and tall split stance. Keep your hips square.

B. Open the arms with the elbows slightly bent. Use the upper back and mid-back muscles to expand your chest. Thumbs point away from each other.

C. Lift the arms without straining your neck. As the arms lift, try to squeeze the inner thighs toward each other like a weak pair of scissors.

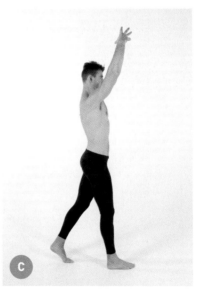

C

3. Woodpecker

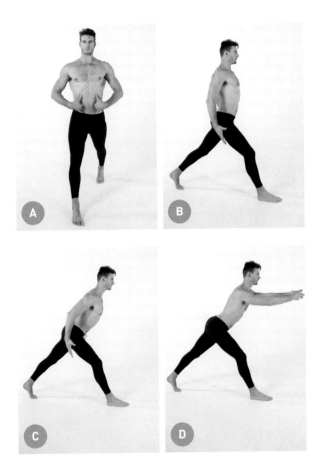

A. Step into a tall split stance with the hips squared and the front knee slightly bent. Take 3 decompression breaths.

B. Open the arms and chest as you hinge the hips back to load the posterior chain of your front leg.

C. Once you feel a stretch and fatigue at the hamstrings and low back respectively, bring your arms forward to counterbalance deeper.

D. Chin back, chest up for 3 to 5 more decompression breaths.

4. Internal Leg Tracing

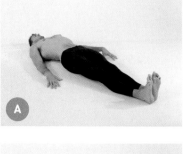

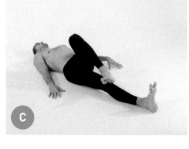

A. Begin in a supine position much like a supine decompression.

B. Lift one leg, internally rotate it from the hip to the big toe and then place that heel on top of the opposite shin.

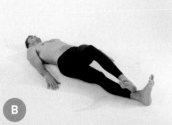

C. Trace the heel of the top leg all the way up the shin until you reach the kneecap or slightly above the kneecap. Maintain internal rotation.

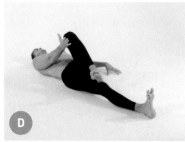

D. Take the opposite hand and press it palm up against the inside of the knee. Ten pounds of pressure should do the trick. The anchoring muscles along the inner leg should begin to fatigue. Maintain the same steady internal rotation as you trace the heel all the way back down the shin and repeat on the other side.

5. Anchored Bridge

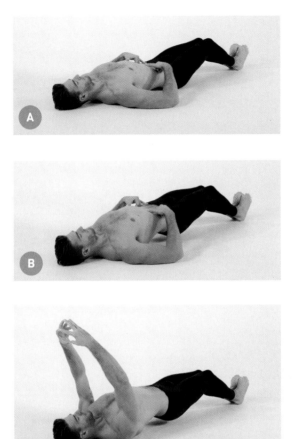

A. Begin supine with legs together and knees bent slightly so that they are not any higher than your chest.

B. Isometrically pull your heels toward your hips without moving them. It feels like the back of the legs activate quickly.

C. Continue pulling the heels toward the hips and squeeze your knees as you lift the hips 1 to three inches off the ground.

6. Anchored Back Extension

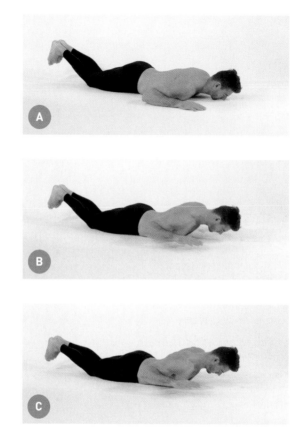

A. Begin prone with knees together and feet a few inches off the ground. The knees remain on the ground.

B. Pull the chin, chest, wrist, and elbows off the ground as you squeeze the knees a bit harder.

C. Take several decompression breaths trying to lengthen your torso with each inhalation. Maintain your height and expansion with each exhalation. Keep the knees together and tight.

7. Kneeling Decompression

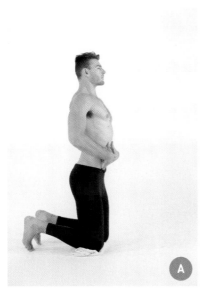

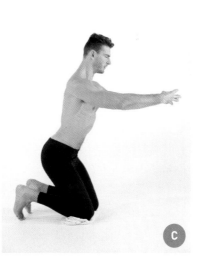

A. If this pose hurts your knees, roll up a mat or a towel. If it still hurts, avoid it. Keep your weight through the knees and lightly touch the floor with your toes. If the toes come off the ground, try to remain balanced. Chin back, chest up.

B. Counterbalance your weight by hinging the hips back and lifting the torso up and forward. Keep the weight through your knees. Keep your feet light.

C. Reach the arms forward as you pull the hips back to add even more resistance to the hip hinge. Stay strong and expand your torso with decompression breaths.

MONDAY, WEDNESDAY, FRIDAY · THREE REPETITIONS OF EACH

TUESDAY. THURSDAY. SATURDAY · THREE REPETITIONS OF EACH

7. Kneeling Decompression

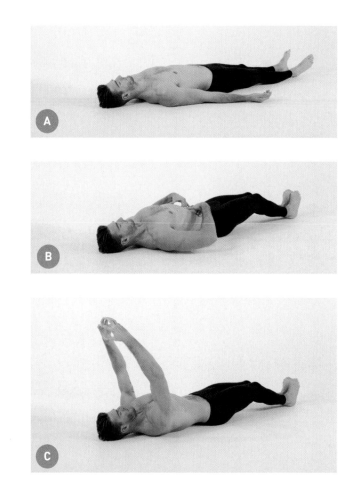

A. Begin in a relaxed supine pose and then bring the feet and knees together. At least toward each other with a steady effort, if you cannot squeeze them together.

B. There should be a subtle bend in your knees, which will help you rotate the hips and thighs toward each other until the groin muscles begin to fatigue. Hold that.

C. Squeeze the upper inner thighs without squeezing your butt muscles. Lift the arms above the chest without straining your neck. Deep breaths will expand your ribcage posteriorly toward the ground.

2. Prone Decompression

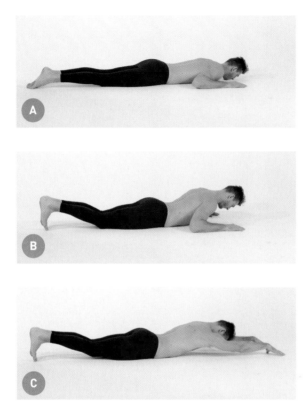

A. Begin in a prone position and bring your feet and legs together. Your toes and knees should remain on the ground for the entire prone decompression exercise.

B. Pull your chin and nose straight away from the floor, do not extend your neck to look upward. Make your neck long and keep your chin back. Reach your arms forward.

C. With the arms forward, as wide as they must be for comfort, press the fingertips to the ground and pull the wrists and elbows away from the ground. Your abdomen, neck, chest, arm, and shoulder muscles should begin to fatigue. This is not a cobra pose or a Superman-type back extension. This pose is to lengthen the spine, not to extend it.

3. Founder

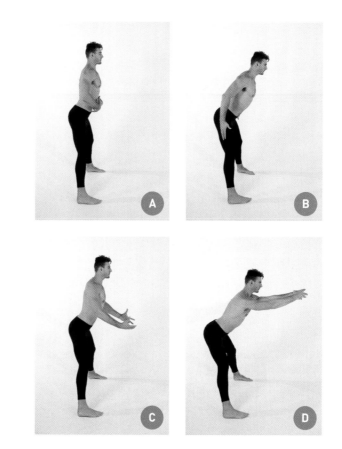

A. Begin in a wide stance with feet firmly pressing toward the ground, take 3 decompression breaths.

B. Open the arms, expand your chest, and hinge your hips back well behind your feet. Allow the knees to gently unlock. The knees must remain above or behind the ankles.

C. Scoop arms forward and up as you hinge the hips farther back.

D. Once you find a challenging counterbalance between the hips and arms, hold the pose for 3 to 5 more decompression breaths.

4. Woodpecker

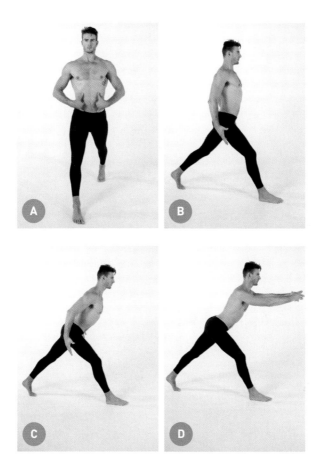

A. Step into a tall split stance with the hips squared and the front knee slightly bent. Take 3 decompression breaths.

B. Open the arms and chest as you hinge the hips back to load the posterior chain of your front leg.

C. Once you feel a stretch and fatigue at the hamstrings and low back respectively, bring your arms forward to counterbalance deeper.

D. Chin back, chest up for 3 to 5 more decompression breaths.

5. Woodpecker Rotation

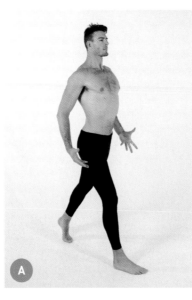

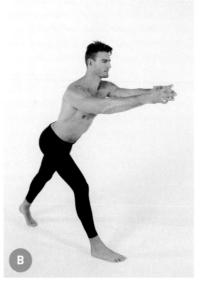

A. Step into a tall split stance with the hips squared and the front knee slightly bent. Take 3 decompression breaths.

B. Open the arms and chest as you hinge the hips back to load the posterior chain of your front leg.

C. Bring the arms forward, load all your weight to the front leg and rotate three to six inches to the same side as the front leg. This should make your glute muscles fatigue quickly.

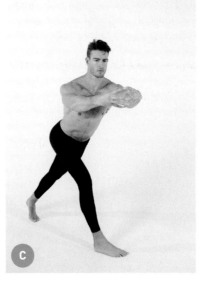

6. Integrated Hinges

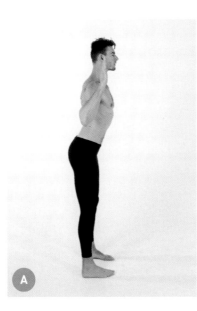

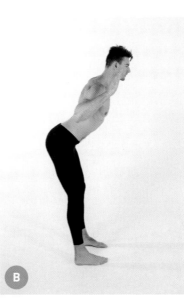

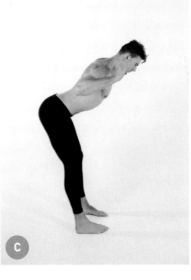

A. Stand tall with legs in any width position you choose—wide, narrow, hip width, shoulder width.

B. Bend your elbows to bring your hands by your ears. This is another chance to keep your chest wide and your back strong as you hinge.

C. Keep your spine long, still, and stable as your hips do all of the work to hinge you back and forth slowly. Try to perform 5 to 10 integrated hinges for each rep.

TUESDAY . THURSDAY . SATURDAY . THREE REPETITIONS OF EACH

Remember to add shoulder tracing into some of the daily exercises as an option as you bring your arms up overhead.

And in addition to this six-day schedule, on any and every day of the week in which you do some prolonged sitting, precede and punctuate the sitting with regular repetitions of seated decompression breathing.

THE SEVENTH DAY

Whatever day of the week your personal seventh day falls on, the aim is to focus on applying patterns of right movement to your activities—and your family's.

If it's your day to garden, for example, concentrate on incorporating kneeling decompression and integrated hinges into your movements.

If you're playing with your kids, keep reminding them to practice decompression breathing while they ride their bikes or shoot baskets.

If you're a weekend warrior out on the sports field/court/body of water/whatever, stay aware of the postures and movements you've practiced over the past six days as rehearsal for today's main event, reminding yourself that the springboard of your power is your pelvis and expanding your ribcage fully to fuel that power.

Even if your seventh day of the week is for brunch and a stroll, take care to inflate your entire ribcage, back as well as front, to make yourself long and strong in the torso, with your chin back, your chest up, space at the back of your skull, and a long, straight line from there down to your tailbone.

THE MOTHER OF ALL WARM-UPS

Make your Foundation Training routine the warm-up for your fitness regimen during these first ninety days—if you can, *in addition to* the

10 or 15 minutes you devote to the daily dose. Whatever your preferred fitness activity is, from aquatics to Zumba through CrossFit or golf, running or weight training, the sequence of that day's daily dose constitutes a warm-up that will switch on the right muscles and switch off the wrong muscles. Most warm-ups simply speed up your heart rate; this one truly primes the body, as a warm-up should, facilitating the activity that will follow.

At the same time, this mother of all warm-ups can help keep your body from slipping back into those postures to which it once complacently adapted.

HOW THE CHANGE TO YOUR BODY HAPPENS

"Consider the postage stamp," someone once said; "it secures success through its ability to stick to one thing till it gets where it's going." Similarly, this initial retraining of your body's foundation depends on your own stick-to-itiveness in repeating the small daily doses. But in the first ninety days of doing so—a mere three months—you will achieve a substantive re-patterning of your body's postures and movements, and you will feel the difference in your own strength and flexibility.

The biggest difference you will notice, however, is likely to be a quicker, sharper sensitivity to the way you are holding yourself or moving at any given moment. As your body adapts itself back into sync with its natural capabilities, it will begin to remind you when you fall back into postures and movements out of sync with those capabilities. Muscles and joints that have begun to readapt to their true purpose and function—the muscles pushing back against gravity to hold you up, the joints serving as hinges of fluid movement—may "notify" you if they are asked to go back to the jobs they complacently adapted to in the past. Hips that have increasingly become your body's fulcrum and the initiator of movement may "complain" if you let your lower back or your legs perform those tasks instead. It's your body telling you that it has begun to readapt to right movement—and that it knows wrong movement when you let it happen.

After ninety days, such readaptation will be well on its way to becoming the new normal—or rather, the old normal back where it belongs—and the postures and movements you have relearned will be well on their way to becoming automatic. And while sticking with the basics of the small daily dose—these fifteen fundamentals of posture and movement—will continue to sustain your body's natural strength and flexibility for a lifetime, you might also want to explore going deeper into Foundation Training practice and expanding your repertoire of movements and combinations.

There are many ways to do this, as you will see when you visit our website at www.foundationtraining.com. There you will find access to video instruction, a schedule of workshops and retreats, contact information for Foundation Training instructors in your area pretty much around the world, opportunities to train as a certified instructor, our blog, and the full complement of social media links.

Why go deeper? One reason is that any form of physical exercise reaches a plateau. We go deeper to push that plateau further out, growing yet stronger and more flexible plateau after plateau after plateau. Another reason to extend outward from the basics of this book is to work on a goal specific to you—for greater facility in a specific sport, perhaps, or for a program of movement specific to your gender, your age, your particular physical strengths or weaknesses.

This book is the substructure of Foundation Training, and the movements it presents can help to keep you naturally strong and flexible for life. But it can also be the starting point for physical training that is more specific, more thorough, and more extensive.

It's not the size of your goals that matters. What matters is remembering the basics—now, later, throughout the day, tomorrow: to lift your torso as you pull your axial skeleton up, support the hip with as many muscles as you can, grip the ground with your feet, widen your ribcage and fill it full with every breath, and in the words of Dr. Tim Brown, my mentor and friend, always to "Stand tall."

Thank you for reading my book.

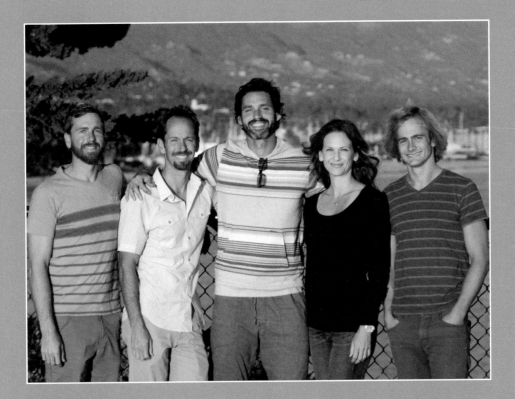

ACKNOWLEDGMENTS

Thank you and you and you.

Foundation Training would have had little chance of succeeding if it were left to me. With that in mind, I would like to thank the extraordinary people who have carried it along with them and put years of their lives into the organization and implementation of our ideas for long-term success. As a team we have helped many thousands of people contend with one of the biggest challenges we face in life, the upkeep of a broken-down body. So much love to Dustin, Brian, Ian, Erin, and everyone else, thank you!

This is a long list:

Karen Rinaldi: Lovely, wonderful, woman, you have been a pillar of truth and guidance for me in an industry that is quite intimidating. I feel like a close friend to you and Joel and an older, hungrier, brother to Rocco and Gio and Vince. There is no way to put everything into words, but know that you were right about business, right about patience, right about life in general. But you should learn to go right more when we surf! I love you dearly, and appreciate every single effort you have put in to seeing Foundation Training come to the surface as a leading theory in health and medicine.

Susanna Margolis: What an amazing writer you are! To take the nonsensical musings of mine, make sense out of them, and then make even more sense out of them is remarkable. This book came to life through your skills, brilliant mind, and pleasant phone voice. Thank you so much, really. This is a dream come true for me.

Dr. Dustin DeRyke: Here we find ourselves thirty-five years old still working and playing together daily. Thank you for your creativity, integrity, support, and friendship over so many years. We've got ourselves a pretty great gig these days! Thank you specifically for the artwork in this book, the anatomy figures, and the general direction in design and look of FT. Unreal what you can come up with.

Ian Silverberg: The only businessman for a business like ours. It has been eye-opening to work with you these past four years. Here's looking forward to many years of a growing community rooted in helping people as efficiently as we can, and a lot of fun along the way. Thank you for giving us young folks a great example to lean toward. A lot of love to Courtney and the kids for loaning us so much of your time too!

Dr. Tim Brown: I've never felt cooler than when I get to hang out, play music, and treat patients with the legend, Dr. Brown. I can remember watching you lecture several years ago, in front of at least a hundred doctors, and smiling as you ended your lecture by saying,

"If you remember one thing from this lecture it should be this book," and you flashed to an image of the original Foundation book. Unreal! Thank you for lending me credibility on tap!

Jeanene Salas: Thank you for love, tolerance, support, food, massages, surf trips, camping, and being a fantastic partner in life, and travel and work and fun. We've got it pretty good!

Dr. Joe Mercola: I'm grateful for our friendship. Your impact on Foundation Training was felt immediately. Your impact in the health community has changed a lot of minds, helped a lot of lives, and advanced a lot of careers, just like mine. Thank you so much for your kindness, support, and inspiration.

Peter Park: The platform you provided between 2009 and 2013 was tremendous. Your work in the strength and conditioning world is next-level, just like your admirable clientele. Through ups and downs and everything else I always value the person you are. A talented athlete, loyal family man, and one hell of a partner in sharing a theory with the world.

Erin Low: Thank you for helping create and implement our absolutely, positively world-class Foundation Training certifications. The four-day certs are the lifeblood of our work and every instructor that we have taught has had a better experience because of your work. You bring so much to FT, you should get a raise . . . Talk to Ian.

Dr. Terry Schroeder: I look back on my internship with you and the year training the USA Men's Water Polo Team as integral growth points in my psyche and confidence. You provided me with such an amazing experience. Thank you.

Dr. "Uncle" Glenn Goodman: You are my initial inspiration toward the health professions. I'm endlessly enthused by your view on life, the effort and energy you place on healing, surfing, loving, and laughing. It's infectious. Now we are even working together, teaching people healthy habits of movement and healthy habits in life. How cool is that!?

Brian King: In five years you've helped me carry Foundation Training to deeper places, better movements, better breathing . . . You have such natural abilities in teaching and educating people to feel what we need them to. I always hope to nurture this ability, to help it grow and see you share your talent more and more with the world.

Kelleen Daugherty: You facilitated Foundation Training in so many ways! Thank you for Ian and Tisha, changing my world for the better forever, and sharing your effervescent kindness with my whole crew.

Tisha Gehringer, Kaeley Christenson, Jenna Dickman: Thanks for being supportive behind the scenes, and also having the ability to remain lighthearted, pleasant, and playful throughout this ongoing adventure of building FT. Your efforts and energy are always appreciated!

Kim Katerba: Thank you for the various efforts you are now putting in on behalf of our main team. I've really enjoyed your presence and feel that bringing you in after you got certified was a great decision for Foundation Training.

Gail DeSart: Thank you for the gentle nudge to patiently form a world-class certification course, and thank you for becoming our first Foundation Training Certified Instructor.

Chad, Sean, Mia, and Shane: thank you for being a part of our world-class Foundation Training certification course and for so kindly sharing an idea you believe in.

Ethan Stewart and Bruno Treves: Thank you for setting the tone of the book, asking effective questions, and putting up with my incessant mind changing. Ethan, you are one of the most talented journalists and wordsmiths I've ever met. Bruno, be patient. As a young, up-and-coming student of meditation, massage, Foundation Training, and so much more, you have so much energy and talent to share, but take your time. Thank you both for the time you put into this project.

Brad and Barbara Goodman: It's a lot of fun growing up and becoming a man around your world. I hit the jackpot in the parent pool, no question about it. Now, five years into the whole thing I get to see you both helping teach Foundation Training workshops and classes, telling all of your friends about it, and even using it on your own every day. It's a great feeling. I love you.

Heather, Ryan, and Teagan Forrest: You are all wonderful. I'm thankful for the opportunity to see so much of you during the past couple of years. Thank you for being stellar examples of a strong relationship, and wonderful humans.

The surfing community: Thank you for becoming early adopters of my work. I swear I've gotten waves just because a few guys in the lineup use Foundation Training. I'm grateful I get to surf, and for the other folks around the world who enjoy and respect the ocean as much or more. Please continue picking up litter at the beach, keeping an eye on other surfers in the water, and having a great time as often as you can!

The medical community: Thank you for having an open mind, trying something new, and recognizing that sometimes the body can become strong enough to heal itself from pretty nasty situations. Foundation Training is blending lines and crossing boundaries. I am so enthusiastic about the use of our work in extremely difficult cases, in all different medical fields. Everyone, go hug your doctors.

To everyone who has offered testimonials, quotes, and support however you have. If you have shared my work with your friends or family or coworkers, please know that I appreciate you. It's been a hell of a ride trying to figure out a way to share this with people.

A special thank you to Martin Reader, Olympic athlete and co-founder of StriveLife Athletics, for acting as our model for *True To Form*.

Last but not least, to my own beat-up and broke-down spine: You sucked at first, but now you're awesome and I appreciate the adversity provided for the last decade or so.

ABOUT THE AUTHOR

DR. ERIC GOODMAN is the creator of Foundation Training and the author of *Foundation*. A graduate of the University of Central Florida, with a bachelors in health sciences and physiology, he earned his doctor of chiropractic at Southern California University of Health Sciences. When he's not traveling around the country teaching Foundation Training, Dr. Goodman lives in Santa Barbara, California.